Praise for *The Ketamine Breakth*

D1106242

"Integrative medicine addresses mind, body, and spirit. The
blueprint provides readers an opportunity for healing th

— **Andrew Weil, M.D.**, #1 *New York Times* best-selling author
of *8 Weeks to Optimal Health*

"Our tools for treating the virtual epidemic of mood disorders, including depression and anxiety, are profoundly limited. The Ketamine Breakthrough *takes us to the leading edge of an exciting, new, and effective approach for these and other mental disorders—a therapy that is so desperately needed. This book provides an empowering revelation not just in terms of the scope of the problem, but also in terms of the promise for recovery."*

— **David Perlmutter, M.D.**, #1 *New York Times* best-selling author,
author of *Drop Acid*, board-certified neurologist

"I highly recommend The Ketamine Breakthrough *for anyone who is looking to target the cause of mental illness at its root."*

— **J.J. Virgin**, *New York Times* best-selling author of *The Virgin Diet*

"Nationally recognized psychotherapist Dr. Mike Dow is always at the forefront of supporting the nation's mental health. The Ketamine Breakthrough *is a must-read for anyone looking for a holistic and integrative approach to mental illness. I give it my highest recommendation."*

— **Anthony Youn, M.D., F.A.C.S.**, America's Holistic Plastic Surgeon®
and author of *The Age Fix*

"Dr. Mike Dow is on the forefront of mental health and this book is 'the' megaphone that will lead this revolution, not only in mental health but health in general. In The Ketamine Breakthrough, *Dr Dow breaks down the barriers and opens the door to improved psychological and physical health. The question is, 'Will you take the first step?'"*

— **Shawn Tassone, M.D., Ph.D.**, America's Holistic Gynecologist and
international best-selling author of *The Hormone Balance Bible*

"The Ketamine Breakthrough is a must-read for forward-thinking people who want to understand and heal the root cause of disease."

— **Kellyann Petrucci, M.S., N.D.**, *New York Times* best-selling author
of *The Bone Broth Diet*

THE KETAMINE BREAKTHROUGH

ALSO BY DR. MIKE DOW

The Sugar Brain Fix: The 28-Day Plan to Quit Craving the Foods That Are Shrinking Your Brain and Expanding Your Waistline*

Your Subconscious Brain Can Change Your Life: Overcome Obstacles, Heal Your Body, and Reach Any Goal with a Revolutionary Technique*

Chicken Soup for the Soul: Think, Act & Be Happy: How to Use Chicken Soup for the Soul Stories to Train Your Brain to Be Your Own Therapist

Heal Your Drained Brain: Naturally Relieve Anxiety, Combat Insomnia, and Balance Your Brain in Just 14 Days*

Healing the Broken Brain: Leading Experts Answer 100 Questions about Stroke Recovery*

The Brain Fog Fix: Reclaim Your Focus, Memory, and Joy in Just 3 Weeks*

*Available from Hay House
Please visit:

Hay House UK: www.hayhouse.co.uk
Hay House USA: www.hayhouse.com®
Hay House Australia: www.hayhouse.com.au
Hay House India: www.hayhouse.co.in

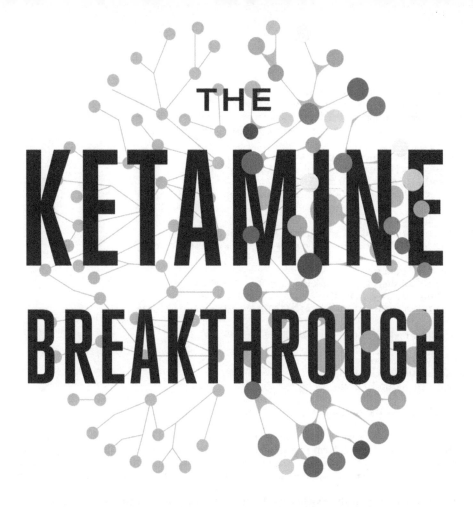

THE
KETAMINE
BREAKTHROUGH

HOW TO FIND FREEDOM FROM DEPRESSION, LIFT ANXIETY AND OPEN UP TO A NEW WORLD OF POSSIBILITIES

DR MIKE DOW AND RONAN LEVY

HAY HOUSE

Carlsbad, California • New York City
London • Sydney • New Delhi

Published in the United Kingdom by:
Hay House UK Ltd, The Sixth Floor, Watson House,
54 Baker Street, London W1U 7BU
Tel: +44 (0)20 3927 7290; Fax: +44 (0)20 3927 7291; www.hayhouse.co.uk

Published in the United States of America by:
Hay House Inc., PO Box 5100, Carlsbad, CA 92018-5100
Tel: (1) 760 431 7695 or (800) 654 5126
Fax: (1) 760 431 6948 or (800) 650 5115; www.hayhouse.com

Published in Australia by:
Hay House Australia Ltd, 18/36 Ralph St, Alexandria NSW 2015
Tel: (61) 2 9669 4299; Fax: (61) 2 9669 4144; www.hayhouse.com.au

Published in India by:
Hay House Publishers India, Muskaan Complex, Plot No.3, B-2,
Vasant Kunj, New Delhi 110 070
Tel: (91) 11 4176 1620; Fax: (91) 11 4176 1630; www.hayhouse.co.in

Indexer: Jay Kreider
Cover design: theBookDesigners
Interior design: Karim J. Garcia

A catalogue record for this book is available from the British Library.

Tradepaper ISBN: 978-1-78817-879-2
E-book ISBN: 978-1-4019-7114-4
Audiobook ISBN: 978-1-4019-7115-1

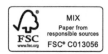

NOTE TO READERS

The intent of this book is only to provide information and the authors' experiences, research, and opinions to readers regarding therapeutic uses of ketamine, which is a Schedule III controlled substance. Ketamine hydrochloride has been approved by the FDA for general anesthesia. Although ketamine has not been specifically approved by the FDA for the treatment of any psychiatric disorders, Spravato, a nasal spray, was approved by the FDA in 2019 for treatment-resistant depression in adults with specifically defined caveats to its usage.

Before embarking on any ketamine treatments discussed in this book, including the Ketamine-Assisted Psychotherapy at Field Trip, a reader should first consult his or her personal medical doctor who would make recommendations based upon the reader's medical and psychological history and current medical or psychological condition.

Readers should also be aware that ketamine should not be used for therapy by individuals with ketamine addictions, pregnant women or nursing mothers, people with a history of psychosis or schizophrenia, active hypomania, or poorly controlled high blood pressure.

The authors and the publisher assume no responsibility whatsoever for any treatments a reader elects to undergo based on any information or opinions contained in this book.

CONTENTS

ACKNOWLEDGMENTS

To the Field Trip physicians, therapists, and staff who are helping us to do this meaningful work, thank you. We go to work knowing that we are changing and, in the case of severe mental illness, even saving lives. *The Ketamine Breakthrough* is a culmination of the thousands of hours of psychedelic-assisted psychotherapy we have provided at our clinics around the world.

To the indigenous peoples, shamans, and healers who have come before us and kept the light and knowledge of psychedelic medicine alive, thank you. We are deeply indebted to you for the wisdom which we have drawn upon.

To the scientists who brought psychedelic-assisted psychotherapy into the west in the 50's, 60's and 70's, thank you. Thank you for publishing and proselytizing—even when it meant risking your reputations, careers, and livelihoods to speak the truth.

To the researchers and clinicians around the world who have made this current wave of psychedelic-assisted psychotherapy possible, thank you. Your work has led to a complete shift in the way we conceptualize and treat health and well-being.

To all those who have directly supported and contributed to this book, we are humbled and grateful, thank you. Reid Tracy, Patty Gift, Sally Mason-Swaab, Margarete Nielsen, Matteo Pistono, David Jahr, Dr. Ben Medrano, Dr. Randy Scharlach, Jeanine Souren, Sabina Pillai, Robin Banister, Joseph del Moral, Hannan Fleiman, Dr. Ryan Yermus, Mujeeb Jafferi, Conrad Page, and Macy Baker.

To the teachers, advisors and muses who have encouraged us to embark on our own healing journeys, thank you. Your inspiration and guidance have been lights in our lives.

To our friends and family members who have endured years of us discussing the minutiae of ketamine-assisted therapy, thank. Your love and support has made this possible.

And most importantly, thank you to all the people who have trusted us to help them on this journey. It requires vulnerability, determination, and bravery, and that's no small ask. May your hero's journeys inspire others to embark on their own.

PREFACE

A Ketamine Breakthrough,
According to the Doctor and the CEO

THE DOCTOR

It's a quiet morning in Austin, Texas. I'm in a room with 30 physicians, therapists, and nurses. My partner, Chris, an emergency room physician, is sitting next to me on the floor. With the colorful yoga mats and meditation blankets all over the room, you'd think we were yogis about to embark on a day of sun salutations. However, any meaningful movement that's about to take place will be with our minds' eyes, not using our limbs. You see, we're a group of health-care professionals who are here to do drugs together. Let me rephrase that—that's what a person who doesn't understand this work would say.

We're actually a group of healers about to collectively embark on a sacred medicine journey. It just so happens that this journey is one of the most effective treatments for depression, anxiety, post-traumatic stress disorder (PTSD), and other mental illnesses. And while we're all here to become trained in, and experience, Ketamine-Assisted Psychotherapy, we're about to discover that every person here has a wound to mend or a life experience to process. And the more this medicine heals us, the more we will have a deep understanding of how we can use it to heal others.

As the training gets underway, I think, *This training isn't at all what I thought it would be.* Instead of daylong lectures and PowerPoint presentations, each day half of us will be therapists as the other half takes the medicine. What I would experience during the week is beyond anything I could have imagined. This surprises me because I came to this training with the bar set high. It was taught by the physician and therapist dyad who had become known as the American pioneers of Ketamine-Assisted Psychotherapy. I had read all of the incredible studies, which, frankly, seemed too good to be true. For example, give suicidal patients a dose of ketamine and most report the suicidal ideation disappears within hours. Ketamine-Assisted Psychotherapy can even help those with the most severe and treatment-resistant depressions who sometimes feel beyond help.

What the research didn't prepare me for was the "ineffable" quality of the journey itself. *Ineffable*: too great or extreme to be expressed or described in words. It really is the best adjective to describe this game-changing protocol. Reading every psychedelic research study you can get your hands on is one thing. Experiencing the death of your ego and a profound connection with all living beings is quite another.

On day one, I'm one of the therapists. We "hold space" for the other half of the group that is taking the medicine today. As the guide who holds space, my job is to help process anything that comes up for the client and help them feel safe and supported. (I soon learn that there's an entirely new lexicon for this work: "hold space" replaces "treat"; "clients" or "journeyers" are preferred over "patients"; "sitter" or "guide" is often used in place of "therapist" or "doctor.") The journeyers don light-blocking eye masks as effervescent music is played loudly through speakers. A spiritual incantation written by a shaman is read out loud as the medicine is given. This is clearly not your average, whitewashed, hospital-based treatment.

As I look around the room, I see just about every reaction imaginable. While most are quiet on this medicine, some are very loud. One physician is laughing hysterically in the corner. At one point, my partner begins moving his arms in an ecstatic fashion. He's smiling and dancing.

Another is clearly reliving a trauma as he shouts out military lingo for all to hear. Some journeyers hold the hands of their sitters and need support throughout the experience; others are completely self-sufficient. Looking at the faces in the room, I would say the most common reaction is one of awe and wonder—which just so happens to be the most effective antidote to depression. As the journey ends, clients begin to make sense of what they saw with their sitter. Like dreams that are quickly forgotten upon waking, it's best to verbalize or write down what you see immediately—so that none of the wisdom is lost or forgotten.

Hours later, we begin to process the experience even more deeply as a group. I'm beginning to understand how beautifully the medicine pairs with therapy.

One physician says that processing the journey helped her to fully forgive her biological mother for giving her up for adoption. The medicine catalyzed a deep healing that had proven elusive for decades. With this one experiential-based aha moment, she would now be able to transcend the one block that was preventing her ongoing work from being truly effective. For most, Ketamine-Assisted Psychotherapy doesn't replace talk therapy; it deepens it. I wondered about this physician, *How many people will she go on to heal in a similarly deep way?*

A woman across the room has a similar story. She had lost her husband suddenly two years earlier and has been in therapy every week since. She talks about how this journey gave her a deep, spiritual knowing that he was okay—something that complemented the more behavioral strategies that talk therapy provided. With joy and lightness written across her face, she says, "I'm actually okay now." Even the military veteran, who looked like his experience was subjectively challenging, reports that his journey was wonderful and healing. Coincidentally, his sitter was a fellow vet who supported him throughout the journey. The deep bond between these two men is palpable. I get chills when he says, "I was okay, because he had my six." He explains that's military lingo for having someone's back. When someone can reexperience trauma while simultaneously feeling safe and supported with their guide, it's pairing the sensory-based memories with a feeling of safety. That can help the brain unlearn trauma responses.

My partner, Chris, talks about one challenging experience that was deeply healing. He was confronted by his claustrophobia in the journey and had to move toward the closing space to confront it. He says his claustrophobia is 90 percent gone (and still does to this day). More importantly, he says the journey helped him to reignite his light that had been dimmed from the stress and trauma of the emergency room. That's what the dancing was all about: his true and most authentic light coming back and moving through his body. This light will help him go on to save countless more lives.

There is a wonderful sense of "I'm not alone" and "I know exactly what you mean" as people nod in agreement and relate to the parts of the journey that were similar. Simultaneously, each journey was unique—and a sense emerges that this medicine brought up what each person individually needed. I have come to learn that Ketamine-Assisted Psychotherapy is often not at all what you think, but it is exactly what your own inner healing intelligence knows you need.

Cut to my experience as a journeyer: After what I have experienced thus far, I have so many feelings about taking the medicine. There's an excited anticipation. Will I have the transformative experience others had? Do I, too, get to experience something profoundly mystical? There is a bit of fear and apprehension. Will my experience be challenging? What if I blurt out something embarrassing? I learn how normal all these questions are when beginning the journey of Ketamine-Assisted Psychotherapy.

After I receive the medicine, I am surprised at how quickly I fall into a dissociative and psychedelic space. It feels far deeper than hypnosis but lighter than general anesthesia. I'm somewhere in between being awake and being asleep. As the lucid dreaming unfolds a few minutes after the injection, there is a moment of stickiness.

It feels like a conversation between my ego and the medicine. Ego: "What's happening?! I've never felt like this before! I'm in control here. I can't let go. What will happen if I do?" Medicine: "It's okay. Trust. Relax. Let go. I'm here to show you something. I promise: This is only temporary. You'll be just fine." Eventually, my ego relinquishes control. I breathe deeply and succumb to the experience. When that happens, there is no separation between "me" as the viewer and everything to be experienced: the flow of music, energy, light, and life.

In this place, I can sense and deeply know the origin and purpose of love itself. Chris's energy is here—but in a spiritual form made up of white and pink light. My wonderful "sitter" (observing therapist) is on the journey with me, too. It's almost like I can see emotions and energies in this space. The abstract becomes seen and heard in a concrete way. If I were to describe where I am, I think I'd call it "the land of love." This land feels like it's the ultimate reality that lies beyond this earthly plane. There is a mother's energy, too. My own mother, all mothers, and Mother Nature are here.

Everyone is in the form of boundless energy. There is something beautiful about not being bound to physical bodies, the containers for our souls. I deeply feel the beauty of connection, the reason sex itself has been programmed as an earthly manifestation of divine love, and why we are meant to form all sorts of interpersonal connections. There is a deep sense that God is Nature, and Nature is God. The separation of science and spirituality does not exist; they are one and the same.

While I had no awareness that I was screaming, I began wailing my partner's name. *"Chrrriiiisss! Chrrriiiss!"* It's more an exclamation of wonder than a cry for help. My sitter soothes and comforts me. Some part of me knows I am safe and supported, which allows me to go deeper and deeper. Unlike ordinary life, there is no analyzing the experience. I am one with it. With no sense of time or space, it simultaneously feels like I'm here for minutes but also days.

And just like that, the end feels like it's coming as quickly as it began. My hands start moving like I am zipping up a coat. Upon integrating and making sense of this journey, I will one day realize that I am "zipping my soul" back into the physical body.

I know instantly that I am forever changed by this experience. As I go back to my daily life, I notice I'm less reactive and more connected. It feels like the result of what I experienced, but there's also clearly a biochemical lift I notice in the days and weeks to come. I call this ketamine's "brain brightening" effects, and for me, the brightening lasts for about six to nine months. This makes sense because ketamine has positive effects on multiple neurotransmitters in the brain. Even when this physiological brain brightening fades, I am relieved to find that some of the most profound benefits are permanent.

By integrating the medicine *and* therapy, it has altered the way I see the world and my place in it. My connection with all living beings is even deeper than it was before this journey began. With that, I know that I am called to bring Ketamine-Assisted Psychotherapy to all those who need it. The path that it has led me down is beautiful, indeed. It has transformed my practice. It includes this book, and if you're now reading these words, it has led me to you.

Dr. Mike Dow

THE CEO

It always starts with the same question.

It doesn't matter if you're having your first psychedelic-assisted therapy experience or are an experienced psychedelic guide. At some point you ask yourself, *When is this going to kick in?*

As a co-founder of one of the world's largest and most recognized psychedelics companies, I found myself asking that exact question right after receiving my first-ever medically supervised and approved dose of ketamine at the Santa Monica location of Field Trip.

Now, if you had asked me as a Canadian kid in high school whether I ever thought I'd find myself in L.A. about to embark on a therapeutic psychedelic experience with ketamine, I'd have laughed at you. And if you had asked my classmates at the time where I'd rank on the scale of "Most Likely to Succeed Because of Changing Attitudes toward Drugs," I'd probably have come dead last.

I would have told you the same thing. Growing up, I was very straight edge toward drugs. While I didn't necessarily object to my friends experimenting with alcohol or cannabis or LSD, they were not for me. The idea of not being in control of my faculties terrified me, a not-so-surprising result of a young childhood defined by the precedent-setting, newspaper-worthy divorce of my parents that led to me living for many years with various forms of police protection at my house to prevent future kidnapping attempts. With such an upbringing, could you blame me for wanting to find some sort of control in my life?

I expressed that need for control, in part, by consciously avoiding situations where I felt out of control, like with drugs and alcohol. Subconsciously, though, I found the control I was looking for by controlling my emotions. At a young age, I made the decision that I wasn't going to let anything get to me. Good or bad, I was a ship that would not be rocked. And it showed. I was even-keeled, monotone, and rarely showed much in the way of emotional response to any situation. I recall, even in my first year of university, one of my residence neighbors seeing this trait in me and making it her mission to get me to scream. (She failed.)

According to many objective measures, this mental strategy of mine worked. I had many friends. I graduated high school with honors, university with high distinction, and was accepted into every law school I applied to. Following law school, I practiced law at one of the most prestigious firms in Canada and then embarked on a career path that had me working in big pharma, for MTV, and ultimately in the world of start-ups.

Every step of the way, my even-keeled strategy worked and worked and worked. Until it didn't.

That day came in late November 2008 when I found myself struggling in a relationship. At the insistence of a good friend, I sought the counsel of Erwin Pearlman, a person who would become my spiritual and emotional teacher (and friend) to this day. While I'll spare you all the details of that conversation, it concluded with Erwin telling me: "The decision to stay, or not stay, in a relationship is fundamentally an emotional decision, Ronan. But you've spent your whole life avoiding feeling and expressing your emotions, believing that you can always think and reason your way through situations. But emotion transcends reason. Trying to think your way out of this situation won't work here. It *can't* work here."

Since then I've been on a journey to rediscover the beautiful, wide-ranging world of emotions. This journey has taken me to many expected—and some very unexpected—places, physically, emotionally, and geographically. Including, once I started learning about the immense psychotherapeutic and spiritual potential of psychedelic compounds such as ketamine, psilocybin, and MDMA, to co-found Field Trip in 2019. It also took me to Santa Monica, California, where I found myself in a zero-gravity chair at a Field Trip location, about to experience my first ketamine-assisted therapy session with the help of Dr. Randy Scharlach, our saga-cious medical director, and Dr. Mike Dow, my amazing co-author of *The Ketamine Breakthrough*.

If you're wondering about the answer to the question I posed in the first para-graph, the answer is: not long.

Within 30 seconds, I noticed the warmth of the ketamine in my lower legs, which then slowly embraced my whole body. It felt like a "letting go," much like that feeling you get just as you drift off to sleep. Shortly thereafter, I found myself expe-riencing something I can only describe as transcendent. I felt like I was witnessing and then forming part of what seemed to be the inner workings of the universe: pure energy, organic and colorful, that was flowing and pulsing and waving in rhythm.

Time surrendered its direction and meaning. What I was experiencing felt like it had always been and would always be. That there was no beginning or end to it. It was pure, essential life. *Eternal*, without trying to import any spiritual or religious meaning to that word.

Many people who have had intense psychedelic experiences describe the feel-ing that everything in the universe is interconnected; that we are all part of a collective source of life and energy; that this notion of "me versus you versus them" is just a false sense of separation, no different from the cells that make up your body. Yes, they are individual cells, but they are still part of your body, they are still part of you.

That sense of being a part of something much larger than myself was what I was experiencing throughout my ketamine experience. It was awe-inspiring.

But it was also unsettling.

As transcendent as the experience was, I also became keenly aware that the intensity of experience at a universal level is far greater than what we experience as people, and certainly orders of magnitude more intense than I had let myself experience through most of my life. And I realized that while the highs of being part of the universe can be infinitely higher than we can imagine, the mundane can also be intensely more mundane than we can imagine.

That was what I was thinking about as the ketamine slowly began to wear off. While ending my first ketamine experience on such an intensely blasé note might seem like a terrible way to reenter this world, I came back with an overwhelming sense of gratitude for everything in my life and just how wonderful and unique it is to be alive, in all aspects of life, the miserable as well as the superb. That feeling of thanksgiving, and the tranquility and serenity that have come along with it, is something that's now stayed with me for months since that experience. It showed me just how much joy and fulfillment I've got in in my life. I just need to keep letting it in.

Ronan Levy, chairman and CEO, Field Trip Health & Wellness Ltd.

INTRODUCTION

Decades from now, we will look back at this moment as the most impactful revolution in mental health since Sigmund Freud gave us psychoanalysis in the late 19th century or the launch of the selective serotonin reuptake inhibitor antidepressants in the 1980s. While the fields of psychiatry and psychology have helped millions cope with their anxieties, depression, and related conditions, today there's an even better, faster, and longer-lasting way to repair the brain and change how we feel.

Prozac is on the way out, and psychedelic-based psychotherapies are rushing in. Antidepressants that mask pain are history. Psychedelics, which immediately lift the depression and anxiety haze while healing the brain in the process, are the future.

Among other psychedelic-assisted psychotherapies, the legal, FDA-approved psychedelic, ketamine, has entered into relevancy, backed by numerous scientific studies and hundreds of anecdotal experiences. The media have caught wind of these developments as *The New York Times* and other outlets have described Ketamine-Assisted Psychotherapy (KAP) as the "most important breakthrough in antidepressant treatment in decades." By combining ketamine and personalized psychotherapy, we can now successfully attend to the brain receptors and neural pathways that cause depression, anxiety, PTSD, and other debilitating conditions. Instead of putting Band-Aids on the brain, we can actually repair the neurological and emotional damage caused by neglect, stress, and abuse.

In this book, we're going to take you through the wonderful, life-changing potential of ketamine: what it is, where it came from, how it works, who it works for, and what to expect. We're going to outline key moments in scientific history that have paved the way for ketamine's future. We'll describe a protocol that we've used for thousands of people with incredible success and answer as many questions as we can so that this will become the go-to resource for anyone considering ketamine therapy.

This book contains hope for those diagnosed with treatment-resistant depression, plagued by trauma, and frozen by fears. It offers a new tool set for people with drug, alcohol, and behavioral addictions; existential depression; grief; and a sense of just feeling stuck. It also gives people with unresolved resentments, anger, and the everyday anxieties of modern life a new path forward. Ketamine can also be an enormously helpful tool to use with couples, groups, and veterans, as you'll learn in this book.

For those interested in the therapeutic benefits of other classes of psychedelics, this book will give you a peek into what is legal, safe, and what might be coming. Beyond ketamine, we are finding scientific and clinical benefits from psilocybin (the active ingredient in "magic mushrooms") and MDMA (3,4-methylenedioxymethamphetamine, commonly referred to as Ecstasy or Molly) as well. But don't confuse the street drug use to what we're doing in a clinical setting. We'll explain the dosages and therapeutic processes that yield true long-term benefits. This is not just an excuse or new way to justify getting high—far from it.

That 1 in 10 Americans over the age of 12 are taking antidepressants tells us we have become a medication nation. We have been duped into being doped up. The facts are most people have to try many different antidepressants until they find one that "works"; that most antidepressants take six to eight weeks before they kick in; that most antidepressants must be taken daily; and that it can be difficult to taper off the drug, which may cause withdrawal symptoms. Along the way with antidepressants, people suffer from numerous undesirable side effects that include weight gain, decreased libido, brain fog, and suicidality.

The worst part is that antidepressants are just that. They are simply *anti-depressing*. They do not address the core behavioral or brain issues that coexist with depression, and are almost never pro-joy, pro-awe, or pro-growth. Research from Oxford University shows that between 46 percent and 71 percent of people on antidepressants will experience "emotional blunting."[1] Another study found that patients on antidepressants reported feeling less empathy for others, and yet another showed they can result in less motivation and drive.[2]

Antidepressants don't solve problems, they just cover them up, and at great cost to quality of life.

But what if depression could be lifted immediately, and for the long term? That's what we can do, right now, with ketamine. The number of treatments vary by person and severity, but typically our clients will receive anywhere from two to six medicine sessions that combine ketamine with psychotherapy—or "talk therapy"—in a 30-day span. Some people may require "maintenance" over time, but almost every client will have some kind of breakthrough. When they make sense of this profound experience with concurrent psychotherapy, the transformative aha moments often change the way they see the world and their lives—and this change often lasts forever.

Ketamine is not a "magic pill." The results that we describe above and throughout this book come from integrating the ketamine experience with psychotherapies such as cognitive behavioral therapy (CBT) and Jungian-based depth psychology. The protocol requires medical practitioners and licensed therapists who understand how to apply the experience from ketamine and translate it into a long-term benefit. It also requires you to work hard, dig deep, and break through your past, anxieties, and depression—but it's worth it.

Our clinical reviews have been nothing short of incredible, with 90 percent of clients reporting a significant improvement—measured by patients' scores before and after treatment. Perhaps the only challenge now is finding ketamine in your area. You can certainly find it at Field Trip centers in many cities and countries, where a number of these protocols have been perfected. And with the launch of Field Trip at Home™, anyone can access this life-saving, life-changing protocol. Whether you are experiencing ketamine at Field Trip or elsewhere, we hope *The Ketamine Breakthrough* delivers everything you need to have a tremendous, transformative experience.

Welcome to a psychedelic renaissance with *The Ketamine Breakthrough*.

Dr. Mike Dow / Ronan Levy

PART I

OPENING YOUR MIND TO KETAMINE

CHAPTER 1

GET TO KNOW KETAMINE

"Am I going to feel [sad] like this forever?"

I used to be happy. But after eight years working the streets as a police officer in Toronto, and 15 years as a firefighter, I became hardened, bitter, and cynical about life. Responding to 911 calls, dealing with death, trauma, and emotionally charged situations taught me to "stuff" my feelings. I felt so alone and scared. I didn't want to end up like my friends who I lost to suicide and destructive behaviors like alcoholism. I wasn't drowning but I felt as though I was circling the drain.

My connection with my family had suffered because I wasn't emotionally available. I would become frustrated and angry with myself. The emotional pain was overwhelming.

After many years, I decided to try ketamine. The experience I had was profound. . . . I felt incredibly relaxed, calm, and at peace when I came out of the treatments an hour or so later. . . . Over the course of six treatments, I felt as though I had a renewed lease on life.

—Mark, actual patient from Field Trip Toronto

One of the most closely held secrets in mental health is that throughout the history of psychiatry and psychology, there has been no single course of treatment guaranteed to help depression, anxiety, addiction, and post-traumatic stress disorder (PTSD)—or just feeling stuck in life. Talk therapy, antidepressants, and anti-anxiety medications are offered on a trial-and-error basis, and more often than not take months or even years before marginal progress is made.

Yet, now there is such a remedy.

Time and time again, we see people who have struggled with depression and anxiety symptoms, having "tried everything," experience the weight of their world lift within minutes of taking ketamine in a medically supervised environment. Depression and anxiety go away. True freedom from PTSD, and answers that allow people to break through their ceilings, are found.

Ketamine is that breakthrough in mental health. It immediately improves mood and regenerates lost neural pathways while creating an opening for therapeutic discussions to take hold. It's fast-acting relief, with long-lasting healing. It's safe, FDA-approved, and about to turn the field of mental health on its head.

Clearly, there is a need for ketamine. One in ten Americans are taking antidepressants presently (that's 18 million people in the U.S., and approximately 300 million worldwide), including about one of every four women ages 40 to 59 in the U.S. Approximately 40 million people fight crippling anxiety, and 15 million people are trying to live with PTSD, which plagues many of our war veterans who average 20 suicides per day in the U.S. alone.

We've opened the book by describing our personal breakthrough experiences with taking ketamine in a therapeutic setting; now we want to introduce you to ketamine's broader applications, pivotal research, key differences from other ketamine purveyors, address safety, and answer fully, "What is ketamine, and what can it do for me?"

WHAT IS KETAMINE?

Though ketamine's place in the public's mind may have derived from its nickname "Special K," and related popularity in the club scene, its primary purpose as an anesthetic has served patients in hospitals and emergency rooms worldwide. In fact, ketamine's safety profile, the ability to preserve breathing and airway reflexes (unlike most other anesthetics), and its worldwide accessibility due to low cost led the World Health Organization (WHO) to declare ketamine an essential medication in 1985.[1]

Ketamine is also the first legal psychedelic-assisted psychotherapy available to people across the modern world. Numerous scientific studies since 2000 have shown ketamine can deliver rapid improvement with symptoms related to depression[2] and has neural regenerative properties.[3] It was approved by the U.S. Food and Drug Administration (FDA) to treat depression in 2019.

But don't be thrown off by the term *psychedelic*. A psychedelic refers to a class of compounds that can induce a heightened mental state that is open to profound discoveries from the subconscious mind—especially when administered by health-care professionals and supported by appropriate therapies.

Ketamine is not considered a "classical" psychedelic because of its widely known purpose as an anesthetic, and because it blocks the glutamate receptor NMDA (N-methyl-D-aspartate), and increases virtually *all* the neurotransmitters. This differs from typical psychedelics, like LSD, psilocybin, mescaline, or 5-MeO-DMT, which focus only on serotonin receptors. However, at appropriate doses, ketamine *can* create a psychedelic experience. This dose, based on factors like age, weight, and history with other psychedelics, is a relatively small dose compared to ketamine's original purpose of anesthesia. We don't want to put people to sleep, which is how ketamine is commonly used in the hospital. Instead we find a dose that wakes up the brain, repairs neurons that have been damaged by stress, and leads to profound insights.

Following a psychedelic experience, new neural pathways are created in the brain that can overlay or redistribute former pathways that lead to negative patterns of behavior. Some clients have even described psychedelic therapies as pressing a reset button on their brains. While there is plenty of research on this topic, and more to come, numerous studies have revealed that the power of ketamine to promote mental wellness and healing may be the result of its ability to temporarily suspend the default mode network (DMN) of the brain.[4]

The DMN is exactly that: what the brain "defaults" to when it's not doing anything. It's also believed to be partially responsible for our ego.[5] Its autonomic functions modulate emotion, thoughts about ourselves and others, memories, and planning. By temporarily disconnecting from the DMN, the brain is allowed a clean slate to try on new ways of thinking, behaving, and being in the world. We will go further in detail about how ketamine works in the brain in Chapter 3.

WHAT CAN KETAMINE DO FOR YOU?

With immediate relief from depression and anxiety, and suspension of the DMN, a significant opportunity for psychotherapy is created. Ketamine-Assisted Psychotherapy (KAP), which is the pairing of a ketamine experience with psychotherapy, creates an opportunity to address many behaviors and conditions while the brain is being healed and, in essence, recalibrated. The result is an incredibly fast-acting and long-lasting modality for depression, anxiety, PTSD, and a variety of other conditions—even when other treatments have failed, such as in the case of treatment-resistant depression.

Combining ketamine with concurrent psychotherapy requires both medical professionals and licensed psychotherapists working side by side throughout the treatments. The insights gained from the ketamine experience are discussed with you and bring subconscious material into the conscious mind—sort of like writing down a dream you had upon waking up.

In psychological terms, KAP helps to integrate the ego with the Self. Swiss psychiatrist Carl Jung defined the *Self* as "the totality of a person's being," which contains both the conscious and unconscious. By integrating the ego and the Self, we move toward balance and wholeness. These moments of integration are often described as "breakthroughs," "lifting the fog," or simply aha moments that have profound and life-changing benefits within the biological, psychological, social, and spiritual frameworks. You might think of it as "synergistic alchemy."

Many people suffer from their conditions for years. With ketamine, meaningful breakthroughs can occur within minutes, and life-changing behavioral modifications can be achieved within three to six therapy sessions.

ALLAYING FEARS

Contrary to its fame as a psychedelic club drug, we want to reiterate that ketamine is an FDA-approved medicine both as an anesthetic and for treatment-resistant depression. It is 100 percent legal for the treatment of mental illness, as long as it is prescribed by a medical professional, and has been widely used in hospital settings, including for children, for more than 60 years. And it's not inherently addictive.

Still, some people fear being too exposed to the "mystical," losing control, or becoming addicted. Although ketamine is not suited for everyone (see pages 9–10), these fears do not materialize for most. By following our recommendations related to the *Preparation*, *Exploration*, and *Integration* sessions, ketamine delivers a safe and therapeutic experience.

The protocol, as explained in more detail in Part III, includes the following sessions:

- *Preparation:* To establish personal therapeutic intentions along with general medical guidance that prepare you for the *Exploration* sessions. This includes your "preflight" instructions.
- *Exploration:* The ketamine is administered by the medical staff while a psychotherapist guides you through the experience. This is the "trip" or "journey."

- **Integration:** "Post-journey" analysis and therapeutic insights discussed and interpreted between the client and therapist.

- **Maintenance:** Some clients enhance and extend the treatment effects by coming back for one or more *Exploration* sessions with *Integration* every 1 to 12 months—depending on the severity of the symptoms.

To further allay fears and assure a therapeutic benefit, we've assembled a comprehensive guide to your KAP experience in Part II, and ways of making the most of ketamine in Part III. In short, every step of the journey described in this book is safe and designed to maximize the therapeutic benefit.

For example, we recommend you and your therapist use the *Preparation* session to identify ways ketamine can elucidate root causes, resentments, and fears that are holding you back from enjoying a mentally and emotionally healthy life. This helps establish the desired intentions for the experience. We also recommend having invocations—or, if you'd like, prayers—prepared, using Dr. Mike's preparation meditation prior to the visit, and discussing any other hesitations prior to your first or any *Exploration* session.

During the *Exploration* session, whether in a clinic or at home, you will receive the ketamine dosing while being monitored, and your experience is guided by a licensed therapist. Learn more about our at-home recommendations in Chapter 7. If you try ketamine as a couple, you may journey together or take turns holding space for each other—with the therapist in the room. To capture the insights gained from the *Exploration* session, we suggest you write down what you experienced with the workbook provided in this book. Then, during the follow-up *Integration* sessions, you and your therapist will work to make sense of your experience, finding connection points that yield therapeutic outcomes. There's more to the protocol and therapeutic recommendations in Part III of the book.

The "setting," or physical surroundings for an experience, is also a major consideration for achieving a therapeutic—and safe—experience. We recommend conducting ketamine in an environment and atmosphere void of any distracting or potentially frightening elements. For example, at Field Trip, the settings are outfitted with soothing color schemes, comfortable couches and chairs, and pleasant flower arrangements and fragrances, along with calming music with rhythms and melodies that complement the moment. Ketamine can amplify the subconscious and sensory perceptions. Thus, a peaceful setting is critical for the experience. Additionally, you should be settled into a beautiful and (ideally) private room and seated comfortably, perhaps in a reclined zero-gravity chair. We like using eyeshades and covering you with sheets and weighted blankets to help create a safety cocoon that embodies comfort. Adding music also facilitates the experience, so we suggest calming instrumentals or sounds that do not distract from what is being experienced. Additionally, you will be supported and monitored the entire time.

After taking ketamine, the actual "trip" can produce a range of feelings as the drug takes your mind deeper within, often leading to experiencing a "letting go" of ego. This can create excitement with anticipation and/or trepidation, both of which subside as the journey unfolds. Although ultimately determined by your doctor or nurse practitioner, many people take comfort in knowing that the dosing we recommend is not solely determined by body weight. We take a person's experience and their comfort level with psychedelics into account. If a person is quite nervous about the experience, we start with a very low dose for the first *Exploration* session and gradually increase the dose.

The way we define the "trip" is any experience that can help you expand your mind from its everyday way of thinking and get an honest look at the way in which you see and make sense of the world, allowing you to uncover aspects of your life or ways of thinking that don't serve you while inviting new ways to connect more deeply to yourself, others, and your environment.

Is ketamine addictive? While some people *can become* addicted to just about anything, including ketamine if taken chronically, we are finding that most people ask for fewer sessions instead of seeking extra sessions. With psychedelics, it's been said that "If you get the message, hang up the phone," meaning that people often find what they need from psychedelic therapies and do not feel the need to repeat the experience often, and the vast majority of our clients find this to be the case with ketamine.

However, as with any drug, there is potential for abuse and harm if not taken safely and under medical supervision. Therefore, we use a thorough intake questionnaire that screens for those who may be predisposed to ketamine addiction due to prior ketamine abuse. Perhaps ironically, some people recovering from alcohol and drug addictions, as well as behavioral addictions to food, gambling, and sex, benefit from ketamine (more on this in Chapter 5). As with any medical treatment, there is a careful consideration that weighs the benefit versus risk for any given patient. Overall, there is little to no evidence to suggest that experiences with psychedelic substances result in long-term addiction or physical harm when taken in a therapeutic setting.

WHO IS KETAMINE FOR?

While the bulk of scientific studies that have been published show that ketamine is effective for treatment-resistant depression and related suicidal ideation, numerous studies also suggest it may be helpful in the treatment of anxiety, PTSD, addiction, dementia, attention deficit hyperactivity disorder (ADHD), anorexia, cluster headaches, and obsessive-compulsive disorder (see Chapter 5). But ketamine can assist with other breakthroughs related to feeling stuck in a rut or a situation due to emotional challenges of everyday life. When it comes to mental health, we find people rarely fit squarely in boxes with one tidy diagnosis—which is why we assess all clients carefully prior to moving forward with ketamine.

Once cleared for takeoff, our ketamine protocol gathers insight from within by helping the mind access the true cause of what's ailing the client. During the follow-up *Integration* sessions, the therapist uses the insights gained from the *Exploration* sessions to home in on specific discussion that the patient's mind will gravitate toward and accept. Additionally, we are finding applications for couples and groups to have significant benefits, as the experience and insights are shared in group therapy settings. We believe there are a wide variety of people who would benefit from this advanced therapy, but there are exceptions. In Chapter 5, we go further into detail about the wide range of conditions to help you determine whether ketamine is for you.

WHO IS KETAMINE *NOT* FOR?

While ketamine can help treat a variety of conditions, we recommend taking great care during the consultation process to ensure a good fit for this therapy. Although the use of ketamine therapy is quite safe for most individuals, there are some conditions that will disqualify you from this treatment. These conditions include, but are not limited to, people with active ketamine addictions, pregnant women and nursing mothers, and individuals with a history of psychosis or schizophrenia, active mania/hypomania, or with poorly controlled hypertension (high blood pressure) or hyperthyroidism. However, people with high blood pressure that is well controlled with medication can sometimes be a fit for ketamine. As a result, your medical team should assess blood pressure prior to ketamine administration. We, of course, also monitor your blood pressure during the *Exploration* sessions.

Below we've listed other Absolute and Relative Contraindications for anyone considering ketamine. If you have one of the conditions listed under Absolute, then ketamine is not right for you. However, if you have a Relative Contraindication, you may still be eligible for ketamine depending on the doctor and therapist recommendations.

Absolute Contraindications (A contraindication is a specific situation in which a drug, procedure, or surgery should not be used because it may be harmful to the person.)

- Allergy or addiction to ketamine

- Recent traumatic brain injury (TBI)

- History of psychosis, schizophrenia, active mania/hypomania and currently experiencing a manic or hypomanic episode

- Nursing mothers (While preliminary research suggests ketamine may be safe for nursing mothers, we currently do not treat nursing mothers at Field Trip. We will reassess this position as more research is published.)

- Poorly controlled hypertension or hyperthyroidism

Relative Contraindications

- Obstructive sleep apnea

- Well-controlled hypertension

- Respiratory issues due to weight

- Medication risks (benzodiazepines, opioids)

- Active substance use or significant past substance abuse

- Personality disorders

- Acute suicidal ideation requiring monitoring for the patient's safety (While depression and related suicidal thoughts can be treated effectively with ketamine, those who are actively considering, planning, or have recently attempted suicide should consider immediate inpatient or hospital-based treatment.)

KETAMINE MEDICAL AND THERAPY REQUIREMENTS

Because ketamine is a prescription medication, all ketamine will require the involvement of a psychiatrist or other medical professional who is permitted to prescribe ketamine. In the U.S., prescribers will be required to have a DEA (Drug Enforcement Administration) license for ketamine. On the psychotherapeutic end, ketamine is breaking new ground with proprietary training for therapists who wish to use it with their clients. This includes ketamine-specific training on various therapeutic techniques that apply.

HOW TO USE THIS BOOK

Whether you are considering ketamine, preparing for your first session, or are in the middle of your therapy, *The Ketamine Breakthrough* has been organized to be a go-to reference. In the upcoming chapters, we will take you on a tour of the history of ketamine, other psychedelics, and how ketamine affects the brain compared with other therapeutic approaches and medications. With this well-rounded understanding, you will have a solid foundation prior to undertaking the ketamine protocol in Part III. Next, we will take a trip through history, examining many of the pivotal moments and research in ketamine's development as a medicine.

CHAPTER 2

THE KETAMINE EVOLUTION

I've been depressed for a long, long time. I'd mask it, shoving traumatic abuses from as far back as my childhood aside, all while pushing myself to do more and more, as a result of my anxiety. I'm pretty sure that's why I had a huge (mental and emotional) crash.

I'd been on different medications since 2006, when my ex-fiancé left me two months before our wedding. Later, I experienced postpartum depression, but the prescribed antidepressants didn't really do anything for me. Finally, enough was enough. I had to take the bull by the horns and do something else. That's when I discovered psychedelics, through a segment on *60 Minutes*.

As a straight-laced kid who went to an arts boarding school in Michigan, I'd never done psychedelics before. But I was willing to try anything.

During my ketamine sessions, I came to some pretty big realizations about my life and past traumas. Yes, there were tears and big emotions, but I was finally facing my true self for the first time. At the start of this journey I never expected to feel like a human again. Today, I know I still have work in front of me, but I'm so much further in my mental health journey than I've ever been.

—Ali, actual patient from Field Trip

Ketamine is a dissociative anesthetic, sedative, pain reliever, anti-anxiety, and neuroprotective agent that was first approved by the FDA in 1970. Although ketamine has been around awhile, its applications, and related research, have evolved significantly in recent decades. Used in doses smaller than its original use as anesthesia, ketamine has demonstrated strong efficacy and safety in the treatment of psychiatric disorders like anxiety and depression, as well as for substance and process addictions. Notably, ketamine is such an old drug that it is now available in generic form around the world.

There is also a new, intranasal form of ketamine called Spravato (esketamine), the patented form of ketamine that received FDA approval for treatment-resistant depression in 2019. Spravato contains only the S-ketamine molecule, whereas ketamine, the one used in Ketamine-Assisted Psychotherapy, is a mixture of both S-ketamine and R-ketamine. While ketamine and Spravato are both effective in treating depression, a 2021 review and analysis of 24 randomized controlled trials found that ketamine's original form was more effective than Spravato.[1] It's also important to note that Spravato must be taken in a doctor's office every one to two weeks and is designed for patients already taking a prescription antidepressant. By removing the R-ketamine molecule and allowing only lower doses, Spravato doesn't provide deep or psychedelic journeys. Thus, it doesn't inherently lend itself to concurrent psychotherapy. On the other hand, Ketamine-Assisted Psychotherapy embraces the dissociative and psychedelic nature of ketamine. Ketamine-Assisted Psychotherapy also provides far more variability in dosing, including high-dose, psychedelic experiences—which is not an option with Spravato. When we refer to the brain-enhancing effects of ketamine in this book, we are referring to ketamine in its original form, containing both S-ketamine and R-ketamine. This distinction is important since research has shown differences in these forms. For example, the authors of a 2012 study found that R-ketamine had a longer-lasting action than S-ketamine,[2] while other studies have found R-ketamine and S-ketamine differ in the way they affect brain cells.[3]

The other medical model of ketamine is the IV ketamine-infusion clinic, which still outnumbers clinics and doctors' offices that provide what we are talking about in this book: Ketamine-Assisted Psychotherapy. Intranasal and IV ketamine are *not* designed to be administered with psychotherapy. Ketamine-Assisted Psychotherapy combines the medicine taken in very deliberate ways with concurrent therapy. We hope that by the time you finish this book, you will have a thorough understanding of why we wholeheartedly believe that ketamine and psychotherapy should be paired.

Ketamine has come a long way. In this chapter, we provide the pharmacological and pharmacotherapy background of ketamine to explain its evolution from an anesthetic to a modern-day mental health marvel.

As mentioned, ketamine is not a typical psychedelic medicine, but can deliver psychedelic experiences. So it's worth noting that psychedelics have been used to create profound and lasting change for thousands of years—often in spiritual or religious ceremonies. Although psychedelics have been common in traditional and some Indigenous spiritual-cultural practices for millennia, their incorporation into modern medical practices has been met with legislative and social hurdles. The unmet and increased need for treatments for neuropsychiatric disorders coupled with the growing body of evidence supporting the efficacy of psychedelics has renewed public and medical interest in psychedelic medicine. Scientists widely agree that psychedelics present promising health benefits and favorable safety profiles compared to illegally and legally consumed drugs, and even many pharmaceutical treatments.

Although the evolution of psychedelics use may deserve its own book, we believe the history of ketamine cannot be fully explained without the broader context of its psychedelic past.

While ketamine is a man-made drug not typically considered to fall into the psychedelic class, the way we apply it—and its related effects—gives us reason to categorize it with other psychedelics like LSD, psilocybin, MDMA (3,4-methylenedioxy-methamphetamine), 5-MeO-DMT, mescaline, or the South American psychoactive brew called ayahuasca. While nobody knows for certain when these psychedelics began to be used for medicinal or spiritual purposes, one scholar suggests psychedelic-laced wine may have been part of both the ritual called "the Mysteries" in ancient Greece and the Eucharist for early Greek-speaking Christians.[4] Indigenous peoples have been using psychedelics in their ceremonies for generations.

As psychedelics continue to be used all over the world to enrich ceremonies and for personal enlightenment, elements of these rituals have likely directly or indirectly influenced ketamine and other psychedelic-assisted psychotherapies. In the table on page 16, notice the similarities and differences of (a) religious/ceremonial use of psychedelics, (b) recreational ketamine use, (c) the use of ketamine to treat depression at IV clinics or intranasal Spravato, and, finally, (d) Ketamine-Assisted Psychotherapy.

Religious/Ceremonial Use of Psychedelics	Recreational Ketamine Use	Medical Ketamine Use for Depression (e.g., IV clinics, intranasal)	Ketamine-Assisted Psychotherapy (KAP)
Sacred and intentional	Not sacred or intentional	Not sacred, possibly intentional	Sacred and intentional
Taken with others: carefully selected indigenous leaders or religious organization	Taken alone or with others; if in a group, the people around you have not been carefully selected (e.g., at a party or club)	Taken with others: carefully selected professionals	Taken with others: carefully selected professionals
Guided by a designated sober guide who is a trained spiritual leader	No designated sober guide or professional	Guided by a physician or nurse who monitors you medically	Guided by both a physician or nurse who monitors you medically and a therapist who supports you psychologically
Usually legal by way of religious protection clauses (e.g., members of churches in the U.S. can take ayahuasca, but illegal for most, etc.) or "gray area" status (e.g., possession has been decriminalized)	Illegal	Legal when prescribed for a diagnosable condition	Legal when prescribed for a diagnosable condition
Preparation required	No preparation required	No preparation required	Preparation required
Integration required	No integration required	No integration required	Integration required
Not medically monitored	Not medically monitored	Medically monitored	Medically monitored
Little/no physical risk	Harm to the liver and bladder documented in high-frequency recreational users	Little/no physical risk	Little/no physical risk
Primary intention is spiritual growth	Primary intention is fun or escape	Primary intention is short- to medium-term symptom relief	Primary intention is deeper understanding and long-term resolution of the roots that are causing the symptoms

Ketamine's journey to becoming a legitimate tool that combines a medicine with psychotherapy to treat mental illness can be traced back to the 1930s when barbiturate-facilitated psychotherapy was used to treat post-traumatic stress.[5] In the 1940s, "narco-analysis" used sedating Pentothal and sodium Amytal, which acted as both truth serum and access point to the subconscious.

Then something revolutionary happened. In 1943, Swiss chemist Albert Hofman discovered a drug he synthesized that had psychedelic properties: LSD (lysergic acid diethylamide). It appeared medicine-assisted psychotherapy would finally make its way into mainstream mental health. In fact, Sandoz Laboratories marketed it under the brand name Delysid, and it was used by psychiatrists to treat mental illness around the world from 1949 to 1966 with remarkable results in treating depression, anxiety, and addiction. Bill Wilson, the co-founder of Alcoholics Anonymous, underwent LSD-assisted psychotherapy in 1956 and reported positive effects. At this time, LSD moved from clinics, where it was intended to be used, to the mainstream. But in this wartime era, hippie culture clashed with the will of the government. LSD became illegal in the U.S. in 1967 and was listed as a Schedule I controlled substance by the United Nations in 1971. The beginning of the American War on Drugs commenced with a speech by President Richard Nixon in 1971.

In the 1970s and 1980s, MDMA-assisted psychotherapy became popular in the U.S. It soon suffered the same fate as LSD and was relegated to the Schedule I list of illegal drugs by the Controlled Substances Act.

After years of psychedelic prohibition, the impressive clinical trials coming out of Johns Hopkins University using psilocybin-assisted psychotherapy marked a major shift and a renaissance of research on psychedelic-assisted psychotherapy. At the time of this writing, psilocybin-assisted psychotherapy is currently only legally available for people as part of research studies in the United States—or in Oregon, which became the first state to legalize psilocybin-assisted psychotherapy in 2023. This treatment is also available at Field Trip's Amsterdam clinic.

While these other psychedelics were subject to a dizzying back-and-forth of public opinion and legality, one has been used every single day in the modern world: ketamine. When ketamine was first discovered, it was used only as anesthesia and analgesic (pain reliever). About a decade after its discovery, ketamine was shown to have antidepressant effects in animal studies. There were a few groundbreaking pioneers using ketamine with psychotherapy beginning in the 1960s. In the 1970s, there was some research noting that recreational ketamine users reported the same effects (some were likely trying to self-medicate their own depression). Since ketamine was being used as an illegal street drug, researchers didn't take this seriously. While there were a few pioneers conducting research and publishing small studies, mainstream medicine didn't really catch on until 2000. That was the year a landmark study found that intravenous ketamine led to fast-acting and profound antidepressant effects in humans.[6] Since then, study after study conducted by prestigious universities and researchers from around the world has replicated those results with the same impressive outcomes, resulting in more than 22,000 published studies on ketamine alone.

KETAMINE PHARMACOLOGICAL TIME LINE

- **1956:** Phencyclidine (PCP) or "angel dust," was the predecessor to ketamine. It was created by chemists at Parke-Davis in Detroit, Michigan. However, it was deemed unfit for human medicine because it caused seizures, neurotoxicity, and hallucinations.

- **1962:** Chemist Calvin L. Stevens, a consultant for Parke-Davis, discovered compound CI-581, which was a next-generational structural analog to PCP. It was one-tenth as potent as PCP and eliminated PCP's problematic side effects. Since CI-581 was a ketone and an amine, it was named ketamine. Ketamine predominantly targets the neurotransmitter glutamate, which is an excitatory messenger that turns on the brain cells and triggers an electrical impulse.

- **1964:** Ketamine was first administered to humans in a trial of 20 subjects. Researchers gradually increased the dose and noted that subjects felt "spaced out" as if they were floating in outer space in subanesthetic doses, which is the equivalent of about one-eighth to one-fourth of a full anesthetic dose; this is the psychedelic state we believe can have therapeutic effects.

- **1966:** The human trial of 1964 became the first human study of ketamine as an anesthetic. The authors discussed how they should write about the strange effects. Initially they wanted to call the dissociative effect *dreaming*, but Parke-Davis didn't like that term; that was too reminiscent of PCP's problematic effects. While talking with his wife, one of the authors said the subjects were "disconnected" from their environment. His wife coined the term *dissociative anesthetic* to describe these unique properties. Unlike most anesthesia that suspends you somewhere between life and death—ketamine, even at high doses, doesn't affect respiratory drive and airway reflexes are preserved, making it a much safer form of anesthesia.

- **1970:** Name-brand Ketalar (generic name: ketamine) was approved by the FDA as an anesthetic for children, adults, and elderly patients. Ketamine was nicknamed "the buddy drug" during the Vietnam War because a soldier could administer it to a fellow soldier if they were wounded in the battlefield.

- **1973:** Ketamine's first reported potential to treat psychological disorders was published but largely went unnoticed for decades.[7]

- **1985:** Ketamine was listed as an essential medicine used for anesthesia and analgesia (pain relief) in adults and children by the World Health Organization (WHO).

- **1989–1992:** Dud pills, which are Ecstasy laced with ketamine, appeared in the rave and club scene.

- **1999:** The United States made ketamine a federally controlled substance in an attempt to stop its illicit use.

KETAMINE-ASSISTED PSYCHOTHERAPY TIMELINE

- **1967:** Salvador Roquet invented "psychosynthesis," involving ketamine and other drugs with individual and family therapy.

- **1970s:** Argentina was an early adopter of KAP. There, it was used with psychotherapy to regress patients back to the womb.

- **1978:** Physician, ketamine fanatic, and isolation tank inventor John C. Lilly, M.D., published *The Scientist: A Novel Autobiography*. Early circles in America began to understand the power of ketamine for psychotherapy and mystical experiences.

- **Late 1990s:** The National Institute of Mental Health, or NIMH—part of the National Institutes of Health (NIH)—began to look at the antidepressant effects of ketamine while searching for treatments more effective than SSRIs.[8]

- **2000:** The first double-blind study using a single IV infusion of ketamine for depression was published.[9]

- **2015:** *Ketamine for Depression* was published by semiretired Australian psychiatrist Stephen J. Hyde. This book made it clear that IV administration of ketamine was unnecessary, noting that oral and intramuscular administration allows for a broader spectrum of dosing and allows for concurrent psychotherapy.

- **2019:** *Science* published an NIMH-funded study finding that ketamine repairs damaged neural activity resulting from stress and depression. It also indicated that dendritic spine regrowth may be a consequence of ketamine-induced rescue of prefrontal cortex circuit activity.[10]

- **2020:** Field Trip opened its first clinic in Toronto.

- **2021:** Field Trip became the first publicly traded company on the Nasdaq offering Ketamine-Assisted Psychotherapy.

Pairing ketamine with psychotherapy was first documented in Mexico by a controversial psychiatrist in 1967 named Salvador Roquet. Influenced by the ceremonies of Indigenous Mexican groups, he called his work "psychosynthesis." As with today's Ketamine-Assisted Psychotherapy, psychosynthesis involved a preparation session just before the medicines were given. But very unlike Ketamine-Assisted Psychotherapy that uses a single medicine at a time, Roquet's psychosynthesis involved combinations of psilocybin, peyote, hallucinogenic morning glory seeds, and ketamine. Unlike the ethereal and soothing Ketamine-Assisted Psychotherapy playlists we use today, Roquet's psychosynthesis was a group treatment that included eight to nine hours of sensory overload. Flashing lights, erratic music, and movie scenes that included sex and violence were played while the patients journeyed in a room together. The patients were then allowed to sleep for a few hours, and then the group integration session began—which would often include family therapy as people were allowed to visit during this time. Roquet used the fast-acting intramuscular delivery of ketamine that we use at Field Trip today. Roquet recommended 10 to 30 monthly sessions as the course of treatment. Despite his somewhat controversial nature, Roquet claimed that 85 percent of patients showed improvement.[11]

In the 1970s, ketamine was used in combination with psychotherapy in Argentina. It was a specific type of therapy that reportedly allowed patients to have a corrective emotional experience by accessing unprocessed material from childhood—which today may be labeled a more spiritual form of psychodynamic psychotherapy. Regression was encouraged with ketamine so that patients could regress back to the womb, die, and be reborn.[12] While this may sound improbable, many clients report a subjective experience of being reborn when given high doses of ketamine. Later in the '70s, ketamine combined with psychotherapy was also used to treat mental illness in Iran. Notably, the research likely helped us realize the therapeutic dose of ketamine in mental health. Doctors there found that 0.2–0.3 milligrams per kilogram of ketamine was ineffective, but 0.7–1.0 milligrams per kilogram as extremely effective when combined with psychotherapy.[13]

In 1985, a Russian psychiatrist named Evgeny Krupitsky began combining ketamine with behavioral psychotherapy to treat addiction. Krupitsky began by combining ketamine with an anxiety-provoking drug to imprint negative associations with alcohol. While many subjects in his research were terrified by this aversion therapy, some had beautiful and ecstatic experiences—with positive outcomes. This led him to pivot to more humanistic, positive types of psychotherapy with ketamine: existential and transpersonal models.

Krupitsky's research was indeed remarkable. Of 111 alcoholic subjects who received his version of ketamine combined with psychotherapy, 69.8 percent were sober a year later versus only 24 percent in the control group. He later used Ketamine-Assisted Psychotherapy to treat heroin and stimulant addiction, obsessive-compulsive disorder (OCD), PTSD, and even some personality disorders.[14] After ketamine became a popular street drug, the Russian government outlawed the use of ketamine for psychotherapy in 2002. Krupitsky's later model is probably the most similar to the modern Ketamine-Assisted Psychotherapy we have developed. Although Krupitsky's program required more hours of preparation psychotherapy than we use, the patients also were administered an intramuscular dose of ketamine, wore eyeshades, and listened to soothing, spiritual music. After journaling the night of their medicine session, the patients would take part in group integration sessions for three to five hours.[15]

In 1994, psychiatrist Eli Kolp began using Ketamine-Assisted Psychotherapy in the United States. Kolp began his career in Russia before moving to the U.S. and, at times, was mentored by Krupitsky. In 1996, the protocol of Ketamine-Assisted Psychotherapy that Kolp used to treat alcoholism was granted an Investigational New Drug (IND) permit by the FDA. After the Department of Veterans Affairs refused to allow him to use facilities to carry out this protocol due to its controversial nature, Kolp transitioned to private practice. His work used KAP for addiction, end-of-life anxiety, depression, and anxiety. Notably, Kolp used the same three-stage format pioneered by Krupitsky, which is also quite similar to our process at Field Trip. Kolp's preparation phase included many of the suggestions we use to enhance Ketamine-Assisted Psychotherapy, such as fasting before treatment, limiting screen time, and avoiding other substances.[16]

Numerous studies have since suggested that incorporating ketamine into psychotherapy may have beneficial effects in many ways, including the following:

- Contributing to the cathartic process

- Stabilizing positive psychological changes

- Enhancing personal growth and self-awareness

- Catalyzing insights into existential problems

- Increasing creative activities

- Broadening spiritual horizons

- Supporting neural regeneration

- Harmonizing relationships with the world and other people

- Reducing suicidal ideation

Forming Field Trip and Taking Ketamine Mainstream

We never set out to make ketamine cool, vogue, or in fashion. After having built one of the largest medical cannabis clinic networks in the world, which became a key part of one of the largest producers of medical cannabis, in 2018 we discovered an opportunity that we believed would revolutionize mental health. We had been introduced to some intriguing science and information about emerging evidence around psilocybin-assisted therapies. Psychedelics hadn't quite made it into the mainstream collective consciousness but our instincts said it would soon, and there was evidence that the global zeitgeist around psychedelics had already shifted. So, as any good entrepreneur would—especially ones who had helped bring medical cannabis to the forefront—we set out to do . . . something.

We started talking to anyone we could. First stop was George Goldsmith, CEO at Compass Pathways, a company leading clinical trials for psilocybin-assisted therapy; he expressed a need for new clinical infrastructure for psychedelic therapies. Next was Rick Doblin, founder of MAPS (the Multidisciplinary Association for Psychedelic Studies), leading clinical trials on MDMA-assisted therapy. Same comment. Then we heard the same from author Michael Pollan and the team at the Beckley Foundation. Everyone was saying the same thing: Build new spaces for psychedelic therapies. The trouble was, in 2018 as today, neither psilocybin nor any other classic psychedelic, was legal. So we were stuck. That was until we learned that ketamine could be legally used like a classic psychedelic and was showing truly transformative potential for people suffering with a host of mental health conditions, from the severe to the everyday.

Armed with a purpose and a direction, Field Trip was born with a mission to heal the sick and better the well through psychedelic therapies. When we announced our existence to the world in April 2019, and opened our first location in Toronto in March 2020, the response we received was overwhelming. The world had been waiting for the moment to arrive, and with the launch of our first location purposely designed for psychedelic-assisted therapies—with a particular emphasis on ketamine—we tapped into a real need.

Since opening, we, along with many other ketamine-assisted therapy companies who are following in our footsteps, have helped countless people find relief from depression, step back from the brink of suicide, and find more joy, wonder, and fulfilment in their lives.

And the world has taken notice. We've been interviewed by, and Field Trip and KAP have been featured in, major media outlets around the world, from *The New York Times* to CNBC, *Cosmopolitan* magazine to *The Hollywood Reporter*, *Popular Science* to *The Economist*.

We always kind of expected this to happen, and now we believe ketamine will lead the way for psychedelic-assisted psychotherapies, and in the process revolutionize the field of mental health as we have known it.

Instead of choosing medication *or* therapy, what if we could integrate all the lessons we've learned from the past about mental health medicine and psychotherapy?

In many ways, that's what Ketamine-Assisted Psychotherapy (KAP) is all about.

Ketamine doesn't replace psychotherapy. In fact, it deepens the process. Instead of spending years in psychoanalysis, what if you could accelerate the process in a handful of ketamine-enhanced sessions over the course of a few weeks? Like Jungian analysis, dreamwork, or hypnosis, ketamine helps reveal past wounds that need to be repaired and reprocessed. It utilizes a non-ordinary state of consciousness to access unprocessed material. Like cognitive behavioral therapy (CBT), it also provides rapid symptom relief and helps people move forward in the present. Therefore, we believe ketamine impacts the "whole person": the psychological, social, and spiritual alongside the biological systems. Ketamine-Assisted Psychotherapy is a revolutionary and effective approach to mental health treatment, bringing medicine and psychotherapy under one roof. In many ways, we're finding it's a truce between the sometimes warring factions of tribalism within mental health medicine *and* psychotherapy.

In this case, the medicine ketamine works on many levels in the brain. For example, ketamine's instant lift of dopamine can improve mood and motivation, which gives us an opening to harness the window of opportunity for therapeutic benefit. Without ketamine, if you give a client with severe depression a cognitive behavioral therapy–based assignment like engaging in productive activities, it's usually hard for them to complete it. But when dopamine lifts instantly, people become more motivated and more insightful. It feels *possible* to do the things that will then help keep depression away in the long term. Ketamine lights the fire, but only you can really keep it burning. That's the beauty of KAP—delivering short-term relief with long-term benefit, utilizing virtually everything we have learned from the past.

CHAPTER 3

HOW KETAMINE WORKS MAGIC IN THE BRAIN

I have dealt with depression and anxiety for most of my life. When my symptoms hit they can include a lack of pleasure and motivation, but it's also a kind of psychic and physical pain. There's a heaviness and tightness in my chest and stomach, or sometimes it feels like a poisonous cloud has taken up residence in my head. I get a feeling like something has happened or is wrong, but it's hard to pinpoint anything specific that causes or justifies these intense, negative feelings.

About 18 years ago, I began taking selective serotonin reuptake inhibitors (SSRIs), which helped for quite a while. But gradually, they were no longer having the effect they once did. I felt really stuck.

I tried a few different things, but nothing really helped. Then my therapist brought up the idea of Ketamine-Assisted Psychotherapy (KAP). A few days later, I started what became one of the most important journeys of my life.

After my ketamine session, I felt a release of some kind, ultimately helping me process and work through my feelings and emotions with the psychotherapist. I find it helps to be proactive and to have a routine with therapy, breathing exercises, and meditation. I also need to eat properly, and I journal when I can. But most significantly, I am no longer on the SSRIs.

I finally feel unblocked. Unblocked in my art, unblocked in my creativity, and unblocked with my mental health.

—*Shay, actual patient of Field Trip*

To fully appreciate ketamine, and how it works magic in the brain, it's helpful to see how mainstream pharmaceutical and psychotherapy treatments have evolved on a separate track from the development of the medicine-assisted psychotherapy you learned about in the last chapter. This backdrop will help you understand just how revolutionary ketamine's effects on the brain are—and how differently it works from today's most popular medications. You'll also see why ketamine is uniquely suited to pair with psychotherapy. We'll review some of the most popular psychotherapy models of the past 100 years, focusing on those that we often integrate with Ketamine-Assisted Psychotherapy.

A DEPRESSING HISTORY OF ANTIDEPRESSANTS IN THE MODERN ERA

In the early decades of the 1900s, dangerous and addictive drugs like opioids, barbiturates, and high-dose stimulants were commonly used to treat depression and other mental illnesses. Symptoms would often subside temporarily, but the resulting side effects were even worse—sometimes causing addiction to the drugs or even death by overdose. Clearly, better options were needed.

In the 1950s, two classes of antidepressants were developed and used as an alternative to the problematic antidepressants of the past: monoamine oxidase inhibitors (MAOIs), which prevent the breakdown of feel-good neurotransmitters like serotonin and dopamine; and tricyclic antidepressants, which prevent the reabsorption of feel-good serotonin and norepinephrine. Benzodiazepines that boost the neurotransmitter GABA (gamma-aminobutyric acid) were invented in this decade as well. While these drugs were less dangerous than barbiturates, they were certainly not without their risks—like drowsiness, sexual function, weight gain, or worsening long-term anxiety in exchange for short-term relief.

Notably, the 1950s also marked the genesis of the monoamine hypothesis. According to this theory, depression and anxiety are the result of low levels of the feel-good monoamine neurotransmitters: serotonin, dopamine, and norepinephrine. While anxiety-relieving, GABA is not a monoamine, but we'll include it under the umbrella of this simplistic theory. Think of your levels of serotonin, dopamine, norepinephrine, and GABA like dials. The theory behind the monoamine hypothesis believes that turning these dials up is the solution to mental illness.

In 1960, the first benzodiazepine was marketed for anxiety. In 1987, the selective serotonin reuptake inhibitor (SSRI) class was born when Prozac was FDA approved. The 1980s also saw dopamine-lifting Wellbutrin receive approval for depression. In the mid-'90s, serotonin-norepinephrine reuptake inhibitors

(SNRIs) were introduced for more severe depression. As the name suggests, this class targets two monoamine neurotransmitters instead of just one. Since then, most of the antidepressants or anti-anxiety drugs people use are one of these four types of medications. They're also used for anxiety, PTSD, and a variety of other mental illnesses.

The popularity and mechanism of these drugs only reinforced the simplistic monoamine hypothesis of the 1950s—which still relies on drugs to turn up the dials on your feel-good chemicals. But this simplistic theory has holes. In fact, research has shown that depleting monoamine neurotransmitters in healthy people does *not* lead to depression.[1] That begs the question, What is the true root cause of mental illness in the brain? There's no simple answer, but we have learned from genetics, trauma, and brain scans about a variety of conditions and how ketamine is often an ideal treatment modality, which we detail further in Chapter 5.

Today, cutting-edge research in mental health is moving away from the monoamine theory—or at least acknowledging that there is far more to healing the brain than just turning a dial on neurotransmitters. As we explain how ketamine works in the brain, you'll see why it has the power to do more than increase or decrease feel-good neurotransmitters, as it repairs the true root causes of mental illness. Ketamine-Assisted Psychotherapy is a functional approach to healing the brain.

A BRIEF HISTORY OF PSYCHOTHERAPY IN THE MODERN ERA

Ketamine's unique effects make it an ideal companion to psychotherapy. By integrating proven psychotherapeutic techniques into the ketamine experience, we can affect long-term change in a person's life. The medicine lights the fire by relieving symptoms virtually immediately; the psychotherapy and associated lifestyle changes keep it burning.

The evolution of psychotherapy has also influenced how we approach Ketamine-Assisted Psychotherapy.

Sigmund Freud coined the term *psychoanalysis* around the turn of the century. A simple way to understand Freudian psychoanalysis is to picture two levels in the mind: the conscious and the unconscious. The goal of psychoanalysis is to make the unconscious conscious.

Then, Swiss psychiatrist Carl Jung broke away from his elder colleague's psychoanalysis when he created analytic psychology, which became a foundation of what's sometimes called depth psychology. Jung believed there was a third level that lies beneath the unconscious: the collective unconscious, containing all the imagery and knowledge every human being is born with. At the time, many of Jung's scientific-minded colleagues shunned this spiritual or even mystical take on the field of psychology. Some scientists still do today. You'll probably recognize many of the terms Jung coined, like *synchronicity, extraversion*, and *introversion*. One of the most popular personality quizzes, the Myers-Briggs Type Indicator, is based on his work. Jung believed dreams were a vital window into the subconscious that could be utilized for deep psychotherapeutic work. The goal of Jungian-based therapy is individuation, a return to the inwardly whole state to reintegrate all parts of ourselves. Ketamine-Assisted Psychotherapy also aims for this wholeness.

In many ways, Jung brought spirituality into the field of mental health. Many of today's popular psychotherapies integrate the subconscious and/or spiritual within their protocols. Like Jungian therapy, Internal Family Systems (IFS) also conceptualizes different parts of the psyche that can be integrated. Dialectical Behavioral Therapy (DBT), Acceptance and Commitment Therapy (ACT), Mindfulness-Based Stress Reduction (MBSR), and Mindfulness-Based Cognitive Therapy (MBCT) all integrate some type of mindfulness or emphasis on the idea that we all have an inner voice or an inner observer that is our real, authentic self.

In many ways, Ketamine-Assisted Psychotherapy's foundation is quite similar to Jungian-based psychotherapy. Jung's humanistic, holistic, and positive view of emotional health is theoretically aligned with KAP. Both are bio-psycho-social-spiritual approaches to mental health. KAP can be thought of as a type of Jungian dreamwork. In a way, ketamine helps the client "dream," and the *Integration* session provides the interpretation of symbols, images, sensory experiences, and archetypes that come up in the session. While some scientists still scoff at the idea of these spiritual concepts, we can tell you that we've seen many clients report and draw strikingly similar themes, symbols, and images after their *Exploration* sessions, and both of us in our personal journeys with ketamine have experienced the same. Whether you believe these universal archetypes and symbols are just projections of a mind under the influence of a medicine or are coming from an even deeper source is up to you—but we find it helpful if people keep an open mind to these concepts.

In 1957, psychiatrist Milton Erickson formed the American Society of Clinical Hypnosis, which still trains health-care professionals in clinical hypnosis today. Like ketamine, hypnosis creates a non-ordinary state of consciousness and focuses on material that lies beneath conscious awareness. Like Jungian theory, there are some controversial aspects—such as hypnosis practitioners who believe they can help clients regress to the womb or access past lives. That being said, the American Society of Clinical Hypnosis teaches Erickson's methods in evidence-based, medically minded ways. Hypnosis and ketamine have even been shown to work synergistically together since they create non-ordinary states of consciousness for healing. Hypnosis can also act as a sort of rehearsal for people preparing to enter the deeper non-ordinary states of consciousness that ketamine can create. Or it can help people go back to the ketamine trance state without medicine. This book contains a script that will help you do both of those things. In the past, PTSD was still called "shell shock," and clinical hypnosis was the treatment du jour used around the world by psychiatrists to treat the condition.

Despite it being less popular today, clinical hypnosis is still remarkably effective for PTSD and other mental illnesses. Recent brain scan studies from research facilities around the world validate the astonishing effects of hypnosis. Interestingly, the clinical hypnosis scripts from decades ago are remarkably similar to the modern "bilateral stimulation" psychotherapies that incorporate left-right bodily stimulation with talk therapy techniques used to treat PTSD today: Eye Movement Desensitization and Reprocessing (EMDR), Accelerated Resolution Therapy (ART), and Subconscious Visualization Technique (SVT). Some advanced practitioners are already integrating these therapies into KAP with great success.

Notably, Freud, Jung, and Erickson all believed that accessing material below conscious awareness and the past was central to growth and healing. They all used their own techniques to access the subconscious and, in Jung's case, the collective unconscious: Freud used psychoanalysis, Jung used dreams, and Erickson used hypnosis. KAP, too, utilizes a non-ordinary state of consciousness to heal. While these psychotherapies promoted a deep understanding of the origins of a person's problems, they were also time-consuming, costly, and hard to measure—since many of these therapies focused on the subjectively experienced world of the patient and a focus on insight and wholeness instead of objectively measured symptom reduction. Psychotherapies that rely on an individual clinician's innate skill and intuition are also inherently harder to study in a scientifically minded way than therapies that use session-by-session treatment manuals.

In the 1960s, the shift away from the subconscious and a focus on the conscious was well underway. Instead of creating non-ordinary states of consciousness, psychotherapy was now about identifying and changing dysfunctional thoughts, feelings, and behaviors. Psychotherapist Albert Ellis published a book detailing his model, Rational Emotive Behavior Therapy (REBT), in 1962. Around that same time, psychoanalytically trained psychiatrist Aaron T. Beck broke with his colleagues when he created cognitive therapy. Beck's cognitive therapy and Ellis's behavioral therapy were the first forms of what we now call Cognitive Behavioral Therapy or CBT, which posits that by changing your negative "automatic" or "irrational" thoughts and actions, you can change the way you feel. In 1977, the first major trial comparing cognitive therapy to antidepressants was published.[2] Therapy was found to be far more effective than antidepressants, or as Beck put it, "People who receive psychotherapy learn something; people on drugs don't." We wonder what Beck would say about ketamine, because unlike someone taking standard antidepressants, clients taking ketamine tend to learn a great deal about themselves.

KETAMINE-ASSISTED PSYCHOTHERAPY: THE BEST OF BOTH WORLDS

Whether they're treated with medication, psychotherapy, or both, there are still so many people who suffer and never find true and lasting healing. If the simple monoamine hypothesis of depression is correct, then why do so many people not respond to antidepressants that "turn up" the dials of their neurotransmitters? Why is the mental illness relapse rate so common—with less than 60 percent of patients experiencing remission with modern antidepressants?[3] Since symptoms return as soon as you stop taking the daily medication, these drugs aren't addressing the damage that leads to depression, anxiety, and PTSD in the first place.

While some forms of psychotherapy tend to be more root-cause oriented than medication, many people with moderate to severe mental illness find that psychotherapy just isn't enough either. As you can tell by Beck's pro-psychotherapy, anti-medication comment above, the modern world has largely separated medication and psychotherapy into opposing camps. Since today's most popular antidepressants are safer than those used in the past, they are often prescribed by primary care physicians or nurse practitioners. And since those practitioners usually don't provide psychotherapy, it often isn't integrated into a person's care. In these cases, medication targets the biology, but the psychological, social, and spiritual aspects of a person are ignored.

Throughout this modern evolution of mainstream mental health, there was a widely used and inexpensive drug right under our noses that can accelerate an opening to access subconscious material, boost neurotransmitters, and repair the brain in the process. While drug companies poured billions of dollars into developing other pharmaceuticals that play with the dials in your brain, ketamine has been available the whole time, being used safely thousands of times a day by anesthesiologists and emergency room physicians around the world.

Since ketamine is both a heart-opening empathogen and an amplifier of the subconscious, it pairs quite nicely with the past-oriented psychotherapies like Jungian-based depth psychology and Ericksonian clinical hypnosis widely used in the first half of the 20th century. Because it rapidly improves mood and dissipates negative thoughts, it also pairs quite nicely with the conscious-mind-focused therapies like CBT that have been more popular in the past 50 years. From a behavioral point of view, ketamine *Exploration* sessions use an inherent form of conditioning since the medicine usually rewards clients for facing their core issues and punishes them when they use defense mechanisms like avoidance to deny them. For example, a client may experience a monster that represents a repressed feeling of shame. In traditional talk therapy, this client could easily choose to avoid talking about this feeling and the related events, which, of course, is more comfortable in the short term—despite any long-term setbacks in terms of growth. In an *Exploration* session, the monster tends to become scarier if the client tries to run away from it. This is because the medicine activates the goals of what we call the Self, the inner parent or the inner healing intelligence as it turns off the defensive parts of the ego that aim to deny or self-medicate. As soon as the client walks toward the dark monster, it tends to transform into an angel or bliss-ful field of flowers. Then, the client and therapist process what this experience means and how it helped to create freedom, acceptance, and the integration of the client's disowned parts in the *Integration* session. The takeaway may sound some-thing like *When I face my darkness, I realize I also have a well of inner strength within me*. Thus, Ketamine-Assisted Psychotherapy is not a polarized choice between medicine *or* psychotherapy. It's not past-focused therapy *or* present-focused ther-apy. It's medicine *with* whole-person-centered psychotherapy—with results that exceed either treatment alone.

Perhaps most exciting, ketamine has *multiple* effects on your brain. We are replacing the unifactorial monoamine hypothesis and its drugs like SSRIs with a *multifactorial* treatment. That's what makes ketamine unique—and why it helps treat conditions like depression and anxiety, even when every other treatment has failed. And when compared to the four other treatments most often used for treatment-resistant depression described below, it's still the only one providing instant relief that people can easily integrate into a modern work schedule with-out requiring general anesthesia and/or surgery.

Transcranial magnetic stimulation (TMS) is an FDA-approved, noninvasive treatment often used for treatment-resistant depression, but like SSRIs, it takes four to six weeks to work for older forms of TMS (involving five short sessions lasting less than an hour per week for four to six weeks) or one week for the newest form of TMS (10 hours per day over five days). Deep brain stimulation (DBS), vagus nerve stimulation (VNS), and electroconvulsive therapy (ECT) are major medical procedures that require anesthesia and include potential side effects such as memory problems, headaches, and seizures. Like SSRIs, these treatments address only the biology of depression if concurrent psychotherapy is not offered. That being said, these four treatments can be life-saving for people with the most severe cases of depression. And they can be combined with Ketamine-Assisted Psychotherapy.

See the figure on the next page, which demonstrates the reduction by more than 50 percent of depression and anxiety in self-reported scores among our clients, even after three months. These results are perhaps even more impressive when you consider the fact that most of our clients have turned to KAP when other treatments have failed. Our outcomes are similar to those of the aforementioned treatments—but require much less of the client's time, without surgery, and focus on all aspects of a person's life that could be contributing to their depression.

Unlike the antidepressants that target feel-good serotonin, norepinephrine, dopamine, or GABA levels at their receptor sites, ketamine begins to work its magic by blocking N-methyl-D-aspartate (NMDA) receptors, which is one type of receptor for the neurotransmitter glutamate. By blocking this receptor, glutamate begins to surge throughout the brain and the hallmark dissociative state begins to set in.

Since glutamate is the most abundant excitatory neurotransmitter in the brain, a cascade of changes take place in the brain as a result—which we'll detail in this section. Because it's such a stimulating neurotransmitter, it has even been referred to as the "juice of the brain." While glutamate is often associated with memory and learning, it also has a profound effect on mood. Today, many scientists are beginning to believe that this glutamate-targeting system may be more central to mood than the ones SSRIs target. Thus, we may finally be moving away from the monoamine hypothesis that's been central to mainstream psychiatry since the 1950s.

HOW KETAMINE COMPARES WITH OTHER MEDICATIONS

Now that you understand how antidepressants are used as "dials" primarily targeting one or two neurotransmitters, let's compare ketamine's multi-action in the brain, which can benefit conditions like depression, anxiety, and PTSD. Notice in the box below how frequently prescribed medications are being used to increase or decrease certain neurotransmitters.

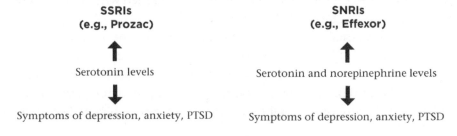

**SSRIs
(e.g., Prozac)**

↑

Serotonin levels

↓

Symptoms of depression, anxiety, PTSD

**SNRIs
(e.g., Effexor)**

↑

Serotonin and norepinephrine levels

↓

Symptoms of depression, anxiety, PTSD

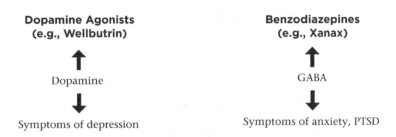

**Dopamine Agonists
(e.g., Wellbutrin)**

↑

Dopamine

↓

Symptoms of depression

**Benzodiazepines
(e.g., Xanax)**

↑

GABA

↓

Symptoms of anxiety, PTSD

Part of ketamine's rapid improvements in mood are because unlike the drugs above, it immediately lifts a feel-good monoamine: dopamine.

RAPID EFFECTS OF KETAMINE

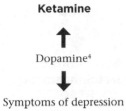

Ketamine

↑

Dopamine[4]

↓

Symptoms of depression

Here's where ketamine really starts to set itself apart from traditional antidepressants: It's a *dirty drug*, an informal term for drugs that bind to many different molecular or receptor targets. While that may sound like a bad thing, it's quite beneficial in treating depression and anxiety. In ways that are still being studied, targeting the neurotransmitter glutamate sets off a domino effect of improvements in other neurotransmitters. This is part of the reason people say that ketamine brightens the brain for weeks. If ketamine is combined with psychotherapy, this brightening can last months after treatment.

Notably, the sustained effects of ketamine via glutamate lift the three neurotransmitters that are the targets of today's most widely used antidepressants and anti-anxiety medications: serotonin, dopamine, and GABA. And it does so without the need for daily dosing and without causing the widely reported side effects of sexual dysfunction, weight gain, or drowsiness associated with traditional medication.

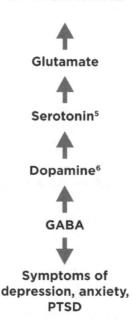

**SUSTAINED EFFECTS
OF KETAMINE**

↑

Glutamate

↑

Serotonin[5]

↑

Dopamine[6]

↑

GABA

↓

**Symptoms of
depression, anxiety,
PTSD**

To sum up, ketamine has been shown to increase several different neurotransmitters. Like SSRI and SNRI antidepressants, ketamine boosts serotonin. Like Wellbutrin, ketamine boosts dopamine. Like benzodiazepines, ketamine boosts GABA. But unlike these traditional drugs, ketamine is just getting started.

Research that has taken place over the past 20 years shows that it works far better than the traditional antidepressants that are most used today. It's like comparing go-karts to Teslas:

TRADITIONAL ANTIDEPRESSANTS	KETAMINE
Target symptoms	Targets root causes
Tend to numb	Tends to awaken
Take weeks to work	Provides relief within hours
Must be taken daily	Has effects that last months
Hard to start and stop	Can be rhythmically integrated at various dosing schedules without difficulty starting or stopping; in other words, it's easy to start or stop
Used as dials on neurotransmitters	Boosts neurotransmitters while simultaneously repairing and growing the brain
Require trial and error to find one that works	Impacts many neurotransmitters, largely eliminating experimentation
Cause troublesome side effects for many	Causes only mild and/or temporary side effects

All this being said, KAP is not an inherently "anti-antidepressant" stance. Every individual case is different, plus we find that KAP can actually make SSRIs work faster and have a synergistic benefit for some people who are already taking them. This is one unique benefit of ketamine over classical psychedelics, since some of them don't pair well with many of today's most popular antidepressants. This is why the initial *Preparation* sessions are critical to assessing the best approach for you.

FIXING AND GROWING THE BRAIN

Let's go back to where the damage in the brain started in the first place. When human beings experience stress, neglect, trauma, or adverse childhood events, it doesn't just deplete feel-good neurotransmitters. These experiences can physically damage brain cells—which is part of the reason experiencing these events increases a person's risk for PTSD, depression, and anxiety. The monoamine hypothesis uses a Band-Aid approach to trauma, which is why SSRI antidepressants are frequently prescribed to reduce survivors' pain and symptoms. In order to keep experiencing relief, you have to keep the Band-Aid on—also known as daily medication.

What if you could replace that Band-Aid with a procedure that could actually fix the damaged organ? Instead of taking the pain away, what if you could undo the physical damage to brain cells that is causing the pain in the first place? That's exactly what ketamine has been shown to do.

In a remarkable study funded by the National Institute of Mental Health (NIMH), researchers used scans to image the brains of mice.[7] Second, they exposed the mice to a stressor in a situation that would mimic abuse or neglect in humans. Third, they imaged the brain again. Sure enough: You could actually see how the stress had physically damaged the cells in the brain. More specifically, the stressor damaged the dendritic spines, which are protrusions in brain cells that receive communication from other brain cells. Of course, effective communication among cells is the essence of healthy brain function and stable moods.

Predictably, the researchers could see that the mice displaying signs of depression had brain cells that had been *physically* damaged. Instead of just low levels of neurotransmitters being the root cause, depression or PTSD can also be the result of brain cells that have been physically damaged.

The fourth step: Researchers gave the mice a single dose of ketamine. Within a matter of hours, they noted behavioral improvements in the mice. In and of itself, this is quite significant. In the fifth and final step of this groundbreaking study, researchers scanned the mice's brains again. Remarkably, they found that the dendritic spines that had been wiped out due to stress had almost instantly been restored.

This study was so revolutionary that Janine Simmons, M.D., Ph.D., at the time the chief of the NIMH Social and Affective Neuroscience Program, said, "Ketamine is the first new antidepressant medication with a novel mechanism of action since the 1980s. Its ability to rapidly decrease suicidal thoughts is already a fundamental breakthrough."

What does this study demonstrate? Well, it helps to explain why ketamine clients experience such remarkable improvements in their well-being. When we use the word *trauma*, we include big "T" traumas like physical abuse and small "t" traumas like divorce. Under this inclusive definition, most of our clients have experienced trauma. We harness the power of the ketamine to fix the brain while psychotherapy techniques help clients reprocess and make sense of these experiences. Ketamine is truly a root-cause solution.

While ketamine helps heal the brain, it can also help *grow* the brain. Many people think of mental illness in ways that are in line with the monoamine hypothesis—needing more of the neurotransmitters that are low. But depression may be more similar to dementia or brain injury than people think. Like dementia, depression and anxiety are also associated with volume loss in the hippocampus, a part of the brain usually associated with memory—but also mood.

The hippocampus also happens to be the part of the brain that is most likely to shrink or grow in an adult brain. On the one hand, it easily shrinks with stress or an unhealthy diet. On the other hand, it's the primary site of neurogenesis in the brain. The catalyst for growth in the brain is a protein called brain-derived neurotrophic factor (BDNF). It's so effective at helping your brain create new cells it's been dubbed "Miracle-Gro for the brain." While most people think of memory when they think of the hippocampus and BDNF, they're also strongly linked with mood. Research has shown that levels of BDNF tend to be lower in people with depression.[8] And the lower the BDNF, the worse the depression tends to be. There are some genetic mutations that lead to lower levels of BDNF, so if you have this mutation and experience trauma, that may be a root-cause source of mental illness. If we can regrow the brain, we can theoretically heal another root cause of mental illness. Could ketamine do that, too?

A 2008 study divided rats into three groups. The rats either received ketamine, a standard antidepressant, or a placebo injection. The rats' behavior was then observed when forced to swim, a popular experiment since helplessness is a symptom of depression. The researchers observed the rats to see how quickly they started swimming. The rats that received either ketamine or the standard antidepressant began swimming more quickly. Researchers dug deeper and measured BDNF levels in the hippocampi of the rats' brains. Here's where ketamine shined: It increased BDNF. The standard antidepressant did not.[9]

In a more recent human study, it appears that this BDNF may even help explain why ketamine is so effective in people with severe, treatment-resistant depression.[10] Subjects were either given ketamine or a sedating benzodiazepine. Four hours later, their depressive symptoms were assessed: A questionnaire was used to measure their subjective experience of mood, and blood was drawn to objectively measure their BDNF levels. The subjects who reported a subjective improvement in mood after ketamine were also more likely to be those with higher objective levels of BDNF in the blood.

So it appears that ketamine is helping to heal another root case of depression by both fixing and growing the brain.

KETAMINE DEACTIVATES THE DEFAULT MODE NETWORK

Now, let's look at how ketamine affects connectivity between different parts of the brain. Because ketamine targets the brain's most abundant excitatory neurotransmitter, parts of the brain begin to connect and disconnect in a myriad of ways. Unlike traditional antidepressants, ketamine profoundly turns down activity in the brain's default mode network (DMN).

What is the DMN? In 2001, a researcher building upon years of brain imaging studies coined the term *default mode* to describe what the brain looked like at rest.[11] In other words, your brain generally defaults back to this mode whenever you're not doing anything. While there are a few exceptions to this rule,[12] the DMN is generally associated with the absence of tasks—which isn't inherently pathological. After all, people can have some pretty good ideas when their minds wander aimlessly.

The DMN also may be akin to what some people mean when they think of the word *ego*. In addition to being a task-negative network, the DMN is the "me, me, me network." Your experience is filtered through a lens of *What does this have to do with me?* There's an inherent awareness of yourself, thinking about yourself in the past through autobiographical memories, and yourself in the future. You can even reference yourself to understand how others may be feeling. Collectively, the DMN is central to one's everyday perception of consciousness.

Problems start to become apparent when the DMN is overactive. Research has shown the DMN is more active in people who are experiencing loneliness[13] and has been linked to rumination and stewing in negative thoughts.[14] With fewer tasks, more worry, and too much ego, it's becoming clear why overactivation of the DMN is linked to mental illness.

If an overactive DMN leads to depression and anxiety, how do we turn it down? Practices that have been deemed "spiritual" or holistic like meditation and acupuncture have been shown to turn down the DMN.[15] Feeling at one with nature can turn down the "me, me, me" and lead to a feeling of "we, we, we" when a spectacular sunset takes you out of yourself for a moment. The cognitive piece of CBT can slowly teach people how to disengage from thinking patterns of personalization and paralysis by analysis, and the behavioral piece of CBT can encourage people to engage in more productive tasks.

Of course, turning down activity in the DMN can take a person weeks, months, or years. There's one way to instantly shut down an overactive DMN: You guessed it—ketamine. Brain scans have shown that administration of ketamine does this instantly.[16]

Since the DMN is associated with an everyday experience of consciousness, it's not surprising that this is one way ketamine is similar to other psychedelics. For example, similar changes in the DMN are seen after administration of psilocybin, the active ingredient found in magic mushrooms.[17]

Having an experience where you lose your sense of "I" or "me" can radically change the way you see yourself and your place in this world. There tends to be more connection and a sense that "all is one."

While difficult to describe in words, anyone who has had a psychedelic experience will have a lasting sense memory of the DMN being turned down. A deeply settled and connected feeling becomes a reference point that can change the way you see your relationship to the world. It's like learning to ride a bike, and ketamine provides the training wheels. Once clients experience ketamine during an *Exploration* session, they can draw a sense of the experience to make other practices more potent. A daily meditation practice becomes easier—and it can become easier to enter those transcendental, mindful states that can otherwise take people years to access. Traditional psychotherapy is helpful here, too. Cognitive behavioral therapy helps to change thought patterns. When paralysis by analysis surfaces, we teach clients to disengage from it and turn off the DMN with purposeful tasks. These everyday techniques prevent the DMN from becoming overactive, and it's yet another way ketamine and psychotherapy integrate in novel ways that heal the brain.

KETAMINE RELIEVES INFLAMMATION

Another root cause of depression, anxiety, and other mental illnesses is inflammation.[18] Short-term inflammation is quite helpful since it's your immune system's second line of defense when the first line of defense like your skin has failed to keep pathogens out. In a healthy body, inflammation is localized and short term. But when this response happens all over the body and brain over the long term, people experience a myriad of symptoms—including cardiovascular disease, bodily pain, and mental illness. Research has shown that people with mental illness are more likely to have markers of systemic inflammation including cytokines, interleukin-6, and C-reactive protein.[19]

This explains why many functional, root-cause-oriented practitioners order labs to measure C-reactive protein: If it's elevated, this may be contributing to or be the root cause of mental illnesses. This also helps us understand why omega-3 supplements or the omega-3-rich Mediterranean diet have been shown to be so effective in relieving depression and anxiety: Omega-3s relieve inflammation in the brain and, thus, improve mood.

Research has shown that ketamine's rapid antidepressant effects may be partially explained by its wide-ranging anti-inflammatory effects.[20] Ketamine has been shown to reduce all three of the anti-inflammatory markers that tend to be high in people with mental illness: C-reactive protein, interleukin 6, and cytokines.[21]

Thus, ketamine has a primary and biological anti-inflammatory effect. When combined with psychotherapy, there also tends to be a secondary, long-term effect since most people will make lifestyle changes that are anti-inflammatory: a better diet, less alcohol, more meditation, and more exercise. And while medicine, food, and supplements are potent anti-inflammatory agents, so is your mindset and the way you think about your place in the world. Research published in 2020 found that cognitive behavioral therapy itself reduces inflammation.[22] So yes, the mind-body connection (or as we like to write, *mindbody*, since they are so very connected) is real.

Now that we've looked back at where ketamine has come from, how it works its magic, and its potential applications, we'd like to share where we believe Ketamine-Assisted Psychotherapy, along with psychedelic-assisted psychotherapy, will likely take us into the coming years.

CHAPTER 4

THE FUTURE OF PSYCHEDELIC-ASSISTED PSYCHOTHERAPY

I'm a former Army Ranger, a husband, and a father of three, and when I heard about ketamine-assisted therapy, I decided it was worth a shot.

When I arrived for my first treatment, I was asked what I wanted from the experience. Well, I wanted to be a better human being. I thought I would get some type of cheat codes to life or an answer on how to be a better human. But the therapy unlocked something even deeper.

Things came out of that therapy that I didn't even think about wanting or needing. I stopped feeling like I needed to drink, and haven't since. I also had mushrooms in the house that went to waste because I felt zero need for them. I'm happier, and enjoying life. People around me felt this shift too. They recognized that I was more present and that I wanted to create memories and better relationships. I'm actually listening and communicating for the first time in a really long time. My wife straight up told me that she wished I'd done this a long time ago. And maybe most importantly, this experience has helped me transform my relationship with my kids.

After my second treatment, I told my two older kids, "You know, I missed a lot of your early lives. Your births. Your first steps. Your birthdays. And I didn't like that. But I didn't realize how much I didn't like that until now. I want to get to know you guys. I want to get to know the little things that make you, you."

My nine-year-old son teared up, looked at me, and said, "I'm happy you're saying that." Today, my relationships with my kids are the best they've ever been.

—*Angel, actual patient from Field Trip*

If at any point you feel as if exploring or embarking on a program with ketamine-assisted therapy is on the fringe of medicine, rest assured. What you're doing is not fringe. Rather, exploring psychedelic-assisted therapies is simply avant-garde, and the future of psychedelic-assisted psychotherapy is bright, full stop. While many researchers and writers like to follow up that statement with something like "although the future of psychedelics is not without challenges legally, medically, culturally, and scientifically," we don't think that caveat is necessary. The trend lines are clear. The science is established. The need is unequivocal. And the cultural mood is not only accepting, it is embracing. In fact, we posit that not only will psychedelics and psychedelic-assisted therapies change how we think about and treat mental health but they will also start to challenge long-held notions of medicine, health, and well-being. They may even start to, in the words of Tim Ferriss, "bend the arc of history" in a positive direction.

Here's how.

Over the coming years, we expect that science will continue to demonstrate the remarkable—and safe—impact psychedelics can have on the brain, the mind, and the body.

Given the remarkable results being generated by the Multidisciplinary Association for Psychedelic Studies (MAPS) in its Phase 3 FDA-approved clinical trials (in which 67 percent of participants who received three MDMA-assisted therapy sessions no longer qualified for a PTSD diagnosis, and 88 percent experienced a clinically meaningful reduction in symptoms with no material adverse events), MDMA-assisted therapy will almost certainly be approved by the FDA for treatment of PTSD by the end of 2023.[1] With two breakthrough therapy clinical trials currently underway for psilocybin-assisted therapy for major depression and/or treatment-resistant depression, it is likely that by the end of 2025 psilocybin will join ketamine and MDMA as safe, effective, and approved treatment options using psychedelics. We expect this trend to continue with companies, including Reunion Neuroscience Inc. (the drug development company born out of Field Trip), working to develop "next generation" psychedelics such as Reunion's RE-104 (a new psychedelic that is very similar to psilocybin but with a shorter trip time) and receiving approval. In other words, in the not-too-distant future, we will have a number of different psychedelics in our toolbox. People working through mental health challenges, along with their psychedelic medicine provider, will be able to tailor individualized programs that speak to that person's unique needs and experiences.

But to start, it's likely that the medical authorization of psychedelics by physicians will be restricted with scrutiny from the FDA and medical colleges overseeing physicians, not dissimilar from what we experienced with medical cannabis. However, in parallel to the regulatory approvals for psychedelics, many states and countries will begin to or continue to move toward legalizing access to psychedelics. (Legalization and regulatory approval have different pathways. Legalization refers to the removal of criminal prohibitions and the establishment of regulated access, similar to what we see happening around the world with cannabis; regulatory approval refers to the FDA, Health Canada, the European Medicines Agency (EMA), or any other government agency responsible for reviewing and approving medicines for specific conditions.)

For example, in the U.S., the state of Oregon legalized the use of psilocybin (Measure 109) in supervised settings with concurrent psychotherapy, which began in February 2023. The Oregon law is significant because the measure went directly to the voters, and the majority of Oregonians said *yes*. In California, the State Assembly is reviewing a bill that would decriminalize psilocybin, as well as MDMA, LSD, and other psychedelics for use with psychotherapy, which would further open the door for statewide acceptance. Laws that allow the use of psychedelics for therapy go beyond merely decriminalizing the possession of psychedelics. If a medicine is just decriminalized, it doesn't mean doctors or clinics can actually obtain it for treatment.

Other states and countries are following similar paths. In fact, as we are writing this book, Canada made psilocybin- and MDMA-assisted therapy available through a Special Access Program to people with serious and life-threatening conditions, including treatment-resistant depression. People will begin to see how strange it is that psychedelics have been illegal while drugs with far more potential for harm and less therapeutic value, like alcohol and nicotine, have largely remained legal. As more business leaders, doctors, and celebrities come out of the "psychedelic closet," it will become normalized.

If you're reading these words on an iPad or listening to them on your iPhone, you may wonder if Steve Jobs's experience with psychedelics helped him invent the device you're now using. After all, he said his psychedelic use was "one of the most important moments in my life. . . . It reinforced my sense of what was important—creating great things instead of making money, putting things back into the stream of history and human consciousness as much as I could."[2] Psychedelics will contribute to people's journey whether they're creating a transformative business or are on a quest for more peace in the world.

As medical and cultural acceptance of psychedelics continues to progress, along with the emergence of a variety of access programs, we anticipate that the medical community will begin utilizing psychedelic-assisted therapies in a manner consistent with what we see happening in "underground" psychedelic therapy today, meaning that doctors and therapists will begin using a variety of different psychedelics paired with therapy as part of an integrative treatment program. While we are not staunchly against practitioners using these medicines under the radar, we are also of the opinion that there will be no need for them to be underground once these medicines become legalized. Of course, spiritual ceremonies in Indigenous groups will continue as they have for generations—since those are already legally protected by religious freedom laws.

In the modern world, legalization and licensing and certification protects both the practitioner and the client. It allows for a code of ethics, malpractice insurance, and insurance reimbursement, and requires continuing education for practitioners. It legally protects confidentiality and makes common-sense ethics mandatory—like strictly forbidding sexual contact with clients. While providers using Ketamine-Assisted Psychotherapy at Field Trip are all licensed professionals, it appears that other medicines in the pipeline will also provide some flexibility in their training requirements—providing a role for "co-sitters" with specific training. For example, the early indications suggest that MDMA-Assisted Psychotherapy will require two people to be present with a client during the experience; one will need to be a licensed psychotherapist and the other can be a "co-sitter" with training in psychedelics, breathwork, yoga, or movement.

Today, training in psychedelic-assisted psychotherapy is not incorporated in the years of education and experience required for psychiatrists, psychotherapists, and psychiatric nurse practitioners. Thus, these practitioners have to have a license first and *then* seek out one of the certificate-based training programs now offered in different forms around the world. When these trainings are integrated into medical school, residencies, and educational requirements, there will be even more practitioners who are qualified to offer these treatments.

While a person may initially seek Ketamine-Assisted Psychotherapy to treat his or her depression, the overseeing physician (who is likely to be a psychiatrist with a preexisting interest or subspecialty in psychedelics, given that most psychedelic-assisted therapies will be performed in specialized clinics such as the Field Trip locations operating across North America) will begin to feel more comfortable recommending, say, MDMA-assisted therapy because they recognize that a significant amount of trauma may be underlying the depression. While not specifically authorized for trauma, short of post-traumatic stress disorder, this off-label use of MDMA or other psychedelics will become more common.

During this time, it is likely that current conventional treatments for mental health conditions will fall out of favor (remember, using bloodletting and leeches was once a well-accepted medical treatment!) as the adaptable, dynamic, and extremely effective and cost-effective psychedelic therapies will offer better outcomes with fewer side effects. As companies realize treatments that target the neurotransmitter glutamate more reliably improve mood than ones that target serotonin, novel medicines that build upon ketamine's mechanism will be approved. These medicines will augment today's Ketamine-Assisted Psychotherapy. While still in the toolbox, Zoloft, Lexapro, and Prozac will no longer make the top 25 list of most prescribed medications. As they move way down on the list, ketamine, synthetic psychedelics, and their derivatives will take their place.

As the utilization of psychedelic-assisted therapies continues to progress, two other trends will emerge. First, science will start to validate psychedelics, because of their anti-inflammatory and neuroregenerative properties. Second, psychedelics will find medical utility outside the treatment of mental health conditions. They will be used in the treatment of central nervous disorders such as migraines and cluster headaches, and neurodegenerative diseases such as Alzheimer's. Clinical trials are already underway to determine whether small doses of LSD are effective in treating this debilitating disease. Other research already includes how and when to use these medicines in cases of brain injury and stroke. The medical community will also start to recognize that psychedelic-assisted therapies not only have application in treating conditions once established, they also have utility in preventing disease. No different than going to the gym to maintain one's physical strength and fitness, people will start to seek out psychedelics for the maintenance of good health, not just the treatment of disease. We foresee a future in which along with one's semiannual dental hygiene appointments, many will begin to schedule semiannual mental hygiene appointments with psychedelic practitioners.

Psychedelics will help us be a true *health*-care system, rather than the "sickcare" system we primarily have today. Being "in treatment" will not mean that something is wrong with you, because if you're still alive, you still have work to do. The process of your growth as a human being continues until your last breath.

This broader embrace of preventive mental health care will emerge concurrently with more and more evidence establishing that our mental and emotional health is tied to basics like gut health and epigenetic tendencies that are inherited but "turned on" by lifestyle. This bio-psycho-social-spiritual shift will have a significant impact on our physical health and well-being. This will end the medical tribalism that pits conventional, allopathic (Western) medicine against functional and integrative medicine models. This peacemaking will mean there will be a greater focus on addressing the root cause, and help prevent other diseases. All practitioners will be somewhat "functional" because they will be armed with methods to help people maximize their well-being. Of course, this will require a huge mindset shift from patients, too. They will realize that for the vast majority of conditions, no doctor can do as much for you as the everyday changes you do for yourself.

An ounce of prevention is worth a pound of cure—which means fewer orange bottles and more green foods. With practitioners who are equipped to understand your mental and physical health on a deep level, and who recommend psychedelic-assisted psychotherapy, even the relationship between physicians and patients will change. These collaborative relationships will improve the quality of life of burned-out health-care workers and stressed-out patients alike.

As more of us consider our overall well-being through the lens of what's possible for our bio-psycho-social-spiritual spectrum—including how to leverage our subconscious and adopt a new relationship to pharmaceutical and psychedelic drugs—change to our health-care system is imminent. Health-care systems and insurance companies will emphasize value-based care where pay is based on how healthy they help people become instead of reimbursing based on the number of procedures done. Our medical system will shift from ensuring that we remain living to helping us be alive.

Psychedelic-assisted psychotherapies are already being used for people with terminal illnesses or in end-of-life care. We will not be afraid of death. Instead, we will talk about it and lean into the spiritual transition. The Western obsession with keeping people alive at any cost no matter how much a person is suffering will be replaced with a compassionate understanding of what it means to live and die. Instead of focusing on *lifespan*, the new focus will be on *healthspan*, the period of one's life during which one is healthy and enjoys a high quality of life. We will manifest a type of well-being that author Tom Robbins calls the "great human adventure," which is "to enlarge the soul, liberate the spirit, and light up the brain."[3]

This kind of evolution takes time. But it all starts here. It all starts with you. It all starts with ketamine. And it all starts as you continue to work through this book.

Now, is ketamine for you and your condition? In the next chapter, we will help you answer that question.

CHAPTER 5

IS KETAMINE FOR YOU?

I've always lived a full and hectic life, which might be an understatement. I suppose when you're forced to live on your own at 15 years old, that's kind of what you have to do in order to provide for yourself and survive. So that's what I did. For years, I threw myself into work. Before COVID hit, I was traveling 200-plus days a year. All of that work led to PTSD, corporate bullying, and anxiety. Along the way, I lost myself and found that I had no sense of purpose or a knowledge of what I even liked. I struggled with alcohol, feeling trapped in a vicious cycle.

When the pandemic hit, it forced me to take stock of where I was in life. Approaching my 50th birthday, I wanted to reset my head, perhaps by traveling to an exotic health retreat that integrated psychedelics. Then a friend referred me to Field Trip and it seemed perfect for what I was looking for.

After the treatments, I've had many realizations and know I won't return to how life used to be. I'm getting back into reading, spending a lot of time with my partner, Christine, and intentionally honoring my personal time as much as business. I'm also looking forward to seeing who I will be at 51, because given everything I've learned in the past year, I now see a ton of potential when I look ahead.

—Patrick, actual patient from Field Trip

Is ketamine right for you?

The short answer to this chapter's question is—most likely. As we've seen, ketamine is a Swiss Army knife kind of medication with a unique ability to amplify virtually every neurotransmitter in the brain while creating an opening for concurrent psychotherapy to take hold. So regardless of the diagnosis you've been tagged with, and even if you don't have a diagnosis, ketamine can deliver a breakthrough in many expected—and unexpected—ways.

In this chapter, we're going to explore the various conditions for which research shows that ketamine can be an effective tool (listed from the most to least common we treat). One thing we know for sure is you are unique, and you may not fit neatly into any of these categories. In fact, in most cases we find that some conditions are actually symptoms of another issue or a combination of two or more. For example, depression can be precipitated by anxiety; an addiction can be a way of self-medicating the hypervigilance we see in PTSD; eating disorders can be a reflection of prior traumas in an effort to attain control that was taken away from you. Still, we want to explain the various conditions to help you zero in on what may be troubling you on a conscious level. This serves to help your doctor with making a diagnosis so you can receive a prescription for ketamine, and will help whomever is taking you through the experience with preparing your protocol. However, we acknowledge that ketamine has a way of revealing underpinnings of problems that may or may not be identified here. That's why we approach each person as a clean slate.

DEPRESSION/SUICIDALITY

Depression is one of the most common, one of the most debilitating, and one of the most undertreated or mistreated mental illnesses in the modern world. It's also one of the most dangerous, as suicidal ideation becomes one of the core identifiers. In essence, people who struggle with depression can't find answers to the feeling of *What's wrong with me?* They may have an internal mantra that things are never going to get better. Typically, *anhedonia*, or the inability to experience pleasure, is present. There's hopelessness, perhaps the most toxic emotion, which even prevents some people from coming to treatment because, they think, *What's the point?*

Depression adds levels of complexity because, again, everyone is different and therefore the source of depression varies. Many people get sent on a medication merry-go-round trying to find something that "works" while absorbing the side effects. (See Chapter 3: "How Ketamine Works Magic in the Brain.") The trial-and-error process can leave a depressed person feeling even worse. But we know, based on experience and the volumes of research on thousands of patients, that ketamine can zero in on symptoms and create an opportunity for long-term progress—even with treatment-resistant depression (TRD) and suicidal ideation.[1]

(Note: Ketamine for depression is not legally available at our Canadian clinics. In Canada, ketamine is approved only for TRD.) This would, of course, make sense since we know that ketamine instantly lifts levels of dopamine—the neurotransmitter of pleasure—while improving neuroplasticity and repairing neurons. Since Ketamine-Assisted Psychotherapy is an outpatient treatment, it is not a good primary treatment solution for people with severe and active suicidal ideation who need hospitalization or inpatient treatment that includes monitoring and round-the-clock care. That being said, Ketamine-Assisted Psychotherapy can be part of a treatment plan for people in this category.

Here are a few studies worth noting:

- A study in mice found that ketamine may be useful in treating depression associated with dementia—and may be especially useful because it has neuroprotective properties.[2]

- Ketamine helped with depression and suicidal ideation in cancer patients.[3]

- With just one dose of ketamine, suicidal thoughts begin to dissipate in as little as 40 minutes and can last 10 days.[4]

- Ketamine may serve instant relief of anhedonia, the inability to experience pleasure.[5]

- Ketamine may also help reduce depression symptoms by improving the microbiota-gut-brain axis, improving the bidirectional communication network between the microbes in the digestive tract and brain.[6]

> *Reflection Question:* Do you have overwhelming feelings of sadness that persist for days, weeks, or months?

ANXIETY

Anxiety is the most searched term on the Internet regarding mental health. It's no wonder, considering the current events, social divisions, and fears proliferating all around us. We also know anxiety can lead to depression, another common condition that is notoriously hard to pinpoint the root causes of but can have dangerous consequences. On the other hand, we do know quite a bit about the nature of anxiety.

Anxiety ranges from episodes of stress to full-on panic attacks, even passing out. Yet stress is a biological response from our sympathetic nervous system that releases the stress hormones adrenaline and cortisol to prepare us to respond appropriately to certain fears. So, stress is totally normal; it helps us survive. Often we refer to stress as generating a "fight, flight, or freeze" response. A more basic definition of anxiety is when you have a sustained feeling of *I'm not okay, and I'm not going to be okay.*

From a more clinical perspective, stress and anxiety are hypervigilant—or startling—responses to real or imagined "catastrophic" fears, causing somatic, or bodily, symptoms. It's a mind-body condition that increases the heart rate, causes sweaty palms, and occupies the individual's thoughts, what we call rumination. Think of the stone-age man who relies on stress when facing the threat of a saber-toothed tiger. The stress can help the man fight or flee. These days, we don't have anxiety like that. However, we can get overly concerned with "what ifs." *What if I get sick? What if I lose my job? What if I lose my house? What if they don't like me? What if everyone stares at me?* and on and on. This would also include anxiety that results from various phobias.

Like addictions, our body and brains can build neural pathways and release neurotransmitters so that these fears, worries, and anxieties become familiar—possibly addictive, in that you can't let them go even though you know they're bad for you.

Ultimately, anxiety is based on fear that becomes crippling to an individual. But the psychosomatic response doesn't equate with the severity of the fear. There's an imbalance between what is real and unreal. Typically, we have found anxiety to be a result of real or imagined fear or trauma from the past that has created polarized thinking, which impacts our experience with fear. This is why ketamine can be an effective treatment, because between the medicine and psychotherapy, we can bring up the scary, isolated, or recurring event(s) and begin to reprocess them in a healthy manner. In cognitive-behavioral-based exposure therapy, the therapist helps the client move toward the feared object to unlearn fear. Sometimes, the ketamine journey is a type of exposure therapy.

With ketamine, we can lift the feelings of anxiety by increasing the GABA and serotonin and turning off the DMN, which gives the therapist time to remodel the memory(ies), resulting in repairing the neural pathways that led to the black-or-white thinking and feelings of imminent doom and gloom.

As with addiction, ketamine improves anxiety by impacting each of the quadrants of the whole person, including the biology of the brain and body, the psychology of our memories, the negative ways it affects our social life, and the disconnection with a spiritual foundation.

Reflection Question: Has stress consumed your mind on a daily basis, to the point that your body ignites a flurry of feelings, thoughts, and/or fears that become debilitating, even harmful to your life?

POST-TRAUMATIC STRESS DISORDER (PTSD)

The Mayo Clinic defines PTSD as "a mental health condition that's triggered by a terrifying event—either experiencing it or witnessing it. Symptoms may include flashbacks, nightmares, and severe anxiety, as well as uncontrollable thoughts about the event. Most people who go through traumatic events may have temporary difficulty adjusting and coping, but with time and good self-care, they usually get better. Symptoms may get worse, last for months or even years, and interfere with your day-to-day functioning." We believe that Ketamine-Assisted Psychotherapy can help people find relief from the "months or even years" of debilitating hypervigilance, fear, self-medication, suicidality, and avoidance that are often associated with PTSD. Although we commonly think of PTSD affecting war veterans, it can haunt anyone who has experienced trauma. Trauma includes big "T" traumatic events like physical and sexual abuse and also little "t" traumatic events like divorce.

Receiving a PTSD diagnosis can be daunting because treatments for this multifactorial and complex condition range the gamut, with no single version hitting the target. Traditional medications like SSRIs only numb the symptoms, and older behavioral therapies required survivors to rehash their trauma over and over again in an attempt to find relief.

Perhaps, until now. Like with addiction, anxiety, and depression, ketamine can peel back the layers of PTSD and rewire parts of the brain involved in problematic fear responses. Ketamine-Assisted Psychotherapy turns down the activity in an overactive amygdala, the brain's smoke detector for danger.

The most recent research backs this up. In 2021, a group of researchers found the first evidence of efficacy for using ketamine to reduce symptom severity in individuals with chronic PTSD,[7] including decreasing suicidality and hopelessness with just one dose. We too have found success using ketamine to treat patients diagnosed with PTSD—so much so that we created a program designed for war veterans called Basecamp, which utilizes ketamine in a group setting. More on this in Chapter 16. We believe the success is due to the protocol that addresses both the biological brain damage and psychological reprocessing.

Also noteworthy is the fact that when treating PTSD with ketamine, we start with lower doses of the medicine to see how the patient reacts. At these doses, there is also more opportunity for concurrent psychotherapy during an *Exploration* session, which can include some of the newer psychotherapy models that treat trauma more easily and fully. Starting with a higher dose could trigger that untreated, unprocessed trauma, bringing back that memory so vividly that it interferes with successful treatment. Each PTSD patient is a case-by-case patient, and going low and slow with the medicine is recommended. Still, we have to face that memory in order to address a therapeutic direction, because in all our work we have to identify where the trauma began and how it started.

> *Reflection Question: Have you experienced a trauma that seems to have lingered in your mind, causing sadness, emotional outbursts, horrifying dreams, feeling on edge, or fears?*

ADDICTION

It may seem counterintuitive to use a drug like ketamine, which can be addictive, to break the cycle of addiction. Yet with ketamine, it's not only possible, it's likely. Care in the screening process must be taken to assure we're not feeding a ketamine addiction. But the fact is that ketamine is a medicine, and when administered appropriately and combined with psychotherapy, it can lead to tremendous breakthroughs in recovery for individuals with addictions.

Keep in mind that in theory, we are all addicted to something or some activity—think of that cup of coffee that is "required" to get the day started, or binge-watching televised programming, or being linked to a mobile device like it's an appendage to monitor social media. Most addictions like these are not necessarily "bad," but they're not healthy either. The question becomes, When does an addiction get to the point that ketamine could be a recommended treatment?

The easy answer is to use ketamine before the addiction causes problems. But generally, addictions are more covert in their control, leading people to believe they don't have a problem until they are overwhelmed with cravings, preoccupied with the drug or activity, and neglect family, friends, and responsibilities in favor of exercising the addiction. Addicted individuals may try to quit after experiencing social, monetary, or even legal consequences, but may not be able to do so on their own.

Addictions fall into two primary categories: chemical addictions and behavioral, or process, addictions. Chemical refers to substances on which the individual becomes physically dependent. Process addictions relate to a mental obsession that stimulates the brain much like drugs can. Gambling and pornography are two common forms of process addictions. Still, people don't wake up one morning and decide, "I'm going to get addicted." It's more likely to be a slow burn that eventually occupies their entire life. Therefore, from a therapeutic perspective the most important thing to consider is that addictions are usually symptoms of unresolved issues, feelings, and mental conditions. This is why, according to science,[8] ketamine can be a powerful treatment modality for addictions. We can get underneath the addiction to expose what led to the addiction in the first place, and layer on psychotherapy to heal the original wounds.

Ketamine may also help reset neurotransmitter levels and patterns of brain activity to a pre-abuse state. These long-term changes in the brain are a major reason why so many addicts and alcoholics relapse. One study showed that ketamine helps prolong abstinence and reduce cravings, pointing to more evidence of how ketamine can be a useful tool in recovery. "Possible mechanisms by which ketamine may work within addiction include: enhancement of neuroplasticity and neurogenesis, disruption of relevant functional neural networks, treating depressive symptoms, blocking reconsolidation of drug-related memories, provoking mystical experiences, and enhancing psychological therapy efficacy."[9]

Additional studies show ketamine lowers relapse rates, helps addicts remain sober, and reduces depression symptoms and cravings.[10]

As to concerns of ketamine addiction, there were two hallmark studies that shed light on this topic. One study, published in 2018, concluded prematurely that when taken together, naltrexone blunted the antidepressant effects of ketamine.[11] Naltrexone is a prescription medication that blocks the effects of opioid receptors and is prescribed for patients in recovery from opioid addiction or alcoholism to curb cravings. This 2018 study was cause for concern, because it suggested that ketamine's antidepressant effects were because it was acting like an opioid—which would make it highly addictive. The next year, a follow-up study using the same design as the one from 2018, disproved those findings, reporting the combination of ketamine and naltrexone was safe, well-tolerated, reduced cravings, and achieved a significant reduction in symptoms of depression.[12]

As you read in Chapter 3, ketamine's magic in the brain has a multitude of effects. If ketamine's effects on depression were due ONLY to the way it targets opioid receptors, it would be cause for concern and a good reason to avoid ketamine. But this is not the primary reason ketamine relieves depression (stimulating glutamate production, boosting neurotransmitters, connectivity, and neurogenesis, etc.). While ketamine has some effects on opioid receptors, it's not the primary reason why it works to improve mood. And for anyone with a history of opioid addiction, the second study suggests that opioid addicts can stay on naltrexone and still receive the benefits from Ketamine-Assisted Psychotherapy—blocking secondary effects on opioid receptors while retaining the medicine's primary antidepressant effects.

Based on this research, and on our own clinical experiences with clients, we know addiction affects the biology of the brain, psychology of behavior, social status, and spiritual foundation. Therefore, we believe ketamine is an ideal therapy for addiction because it can help in each of these areas of the whole person.

> *Reflection Question:* Do you revert to alcohol, a substance, or an activity on a daily basis to help you "deal" with problems, feelings, anxiety, depression, or other issues in order to feel "normal" or avoid them altogether?

BIPOLAR DISORDER

Bipolar disorder comes in two categories; bipolar I and bipolar II. Like major depression, bipolar is a "polar" mood disorder because it oscillates between episodes of depression and a return to baseline. Unlike depression, bipolar disorder also oscillates upward to manic episodes (in bipolar I) and upward to less severe hypomanic episodes (in bipolar II). While we cannot categorically claim that ketamine is an ideal treatment for all people with bipolar disorder, we do believe that in some cases it can have as powerful an effect as it does on depression. Since ketamine tends to be an activating antidepressant by increasing dopamine, which is ideal in lifting people out of depressive episodes, it also can push people with uncontrolled bipolar disorder into mania or hypomania. The most important caution is to avoid ketamine if someone is already in a manic or hypomanic state. Ketamine-Assisted Psychotherapy is often used for people with bipolar II disorder and, with even more caution, can sometimes be used to treat bipolar I disorder.

As mentioned, we approach every client in a personal, customized way. First, we screen for the presence of mania and then we take great care in determining the right ketamine dosage. The good news is that bipolar has similar symptoms and brain dynamics as depression, and remember: Both disorders include depressive episodes.

> *Reflection Question: Do you find depression to include mood swings that range from one extreme to another—including lows but also highs that negatively affect your life?*

OBSESSIVE-COMPULSIVE DISORDER (OCD)

Although we do not know the exact causes of OCD, we do know it shares traits with other conditions related to obsessive thoughts and compulsive behaviors. These include anxiety, depression, eating disorders, and substance abuse, for example. Treating OCD usually uses SSRIs and CBT-based psychotherapy, which requires a long process. With fast-acting relief and the potential for long-term effectiveness, ketamine appears to be a hopeful treatment. Although more research is needed, there is mounting evidence that makes us optimistic about ketamine's potential.[13]

People with OCD often present an uncontrollable urge to repeat a behavior over and over or check and double-check that all things are in order. It can be like a preemptive defense mechanism against a particular, or various, catastrophic fears.

However, ketamine has the ability to put those thoughts and compulsions on hold while psychotherapy helps redefine the reality of the fears, giving patients thoughts and patterns of behavior that actually might help. For example, let's say a person is checking their door lock eight times every time they go out the door. They have developed a neural pathway that has become familiar, and somehow hopeful, in their fear against being robbed. They are trading short-term comfort by checking the lock at the expense of long-term consequences in their life. With ketamine, feel-good neurotransmitters are lifted, which can provide a window of opportunity to use CBT-based therapy assignments. On a deeper level, a mystical experience and a feeling that "all is one" can shift perspectives. In a ketamine journey, the medicine tends to use a form of conditioning and rewards a person for shedding safety behaviors and avoidance.

> *Reflection Question:* Do you get "locked" on a thought or fear, and/or repeat a behavior or ritual so often that it interrupts your quality of life and relationships?

EATING DISORDERS

Eating disorders, of which there are three—anorexia, bulimia, and binge eating—are complex conditions marked by a profound lack of self-love, often perfectionism, and combined with a dangerous relationship with food. Often, there is a history of trauma. Food becomes a compulsive release valve, like a process addiction, or it can be feared to the point of starvation. There is a mixed bag of symptoms and related causes, making eating disorders difficult to treat. In the most significant study using ketamine and psychotherapy for eating disorders,[14] researchers found 9 of the 15 participants in the study responded positively, returning their body weight to acceptable levels. The nonresponders were those who did not take the concurrent psychotherapy seriously, so meaningful changes were not achieved.

Although more research is needed, we believe ketamine can be extremely helpful with eating disorders because of the way it disconnects the DMN while surfacing the root causes for the behavior. By adding psychotherapy, we can help patients enhance self-esteem, begin new habits that demonstrate love for themselves, and create a new relationship with food. Ketamine-Assisted Psychotherapy is not a suitable primary treatment for anorexia, which can be life-threatening and requires inpatient care. It can, however, be a part of a person's treatment plan when he or she is physically stable.

> *Reflection Question:* Do you have a problematic relationship with food?

PAIN AND CHRONIC CONDITIONS

Since 1970, ketamine has been used in hospitals as a sedative and pain-relieving analgesic, so we know ketamine can directly help with pain. While IV ketamine clinics focus on the pain itself, Ketamine-Assisted Psychotherapy aims to change a person's relationship to pain—in the same way mindfulness or prescription antidepressants can be helpful by addressing pain in an indirect way.

By changing this relationship, we have found Ketamine-Assisted Psychotherapy to be a helpful adjunct to chronic or hard-to-treat conditions/syndromes like auto-immune diseases, chronic Lyme disease, fibromyalgia, migraines, polycystic ovary syndrome, pelvic pain, chronic fatigue syndrome, and terminal illness. When someone has any of these conditions, it usually leads to depression or anxiety about the condition. If we can ease or shift the mindset about the pain or condition, the subjective experience of pain often improves. Sometimes a trauma is uncovered that has a direct or indirect relationship to pain or a condition. Other times, the mystical experience of an *Exploration* session provides a powerful reframe.

Pain itself is often a result of inflammation. One study concluded, "ketamine appears as a unique 'homeostatic regulator' of the acute inflammatory reaction and the stress-induced immune disturbances."[15] Pain from (refractory chronic) migraine headaches is also historically difficult to treat. However, one study found that all the patients who received ketamine reported significant improvement in pain symptoms.[16] However, ketamine is not a preferred alternative for pain from "normal" or benign headaches.[17]

By using a whole-person-centered treatment like Ketamine-Assisted Psychotherapy, we may be able to treat both mind and body. While it's not a panacea, we encourage people who fall into this category to consider Ketamine-Assisted Psychotherapy. Our staff can assess you on an individual basis to determine whether ketamine is a possible fit.

While ketamine is not intended to be a long-term remedy for chronic pain, we have seen it help some people indirectly.

Reflection Question: Is your relationship to pain or a condition negatively and profoundly affecting your mood and your life?

NON-DIAGNOSIS

Before addressing the various conditions that follow in alphabetical order, let's start with people who don't have a diagnosis in mind but feel stuck in life. Something is holding them back, but they just can't put a finger on "it." In each of our own personal cases, we didn't have a condition but wanted to attain a higher level of consciousness. In the process, we both discovered something new about ourselves that gave us clarity about pursuing the best we can be.

The truth is, you may not know what is troubling you. It could be unresolved grief, a repressed trauma, or feelings of low self-worth from a divorce or other major event. You may have resentments or fears that have been too difficult to face and hold you back from being able to trust and maintain safe relationships. You may have a genetic predisposition that has not been identified, or you experienced neglect and abandonment as a child, which is creeping into your ability to feel fulfilled.

Here's an example of a real-life scenario. A client came in after going through a difficult divorce. While we initially found that he met the criteria for a minor diagnosis, his primary problem was a complete inability to move on after the divorce. During his *Exploration* sessions, he discovered that there was a lifetime full of repressed abuse memories, low self-worth, several dysfunctional relationships, and other disastrous childhood experiences that had been unresolved for 45 years! He didn't fit into a box, but he definitely needed a breakthrough, which ketamine delivered like a heat-seeking missile.

Classically, these undefined diagnoses would fall under the "adjustment disorder" category, however it's a catchall category to fit the paradigm of the medical system and isn't always 100 percent reflective of what's really in the way. Neither are "major" diagnoses like major depressive disorder. The diagnoses tell you *what* you have but do little to help explain *why* you're feeling this way. But it will help you get a prescription, if you fit this blurry, non-diagnosis category. Answer the question below to help identify whether this fits you.

> *Reflection Question: Do you have a strong sense that you need something different in your life, or that something is holding you back, even if you don't know exactly what that is?*

If you answered "Yes" to any of the Reflection Questions, you may have a reason to explore ketamine further with your doctor or with us at Field Trip. We know ketamine has tremendous potential with the conditions cited in this chapter, and we are seeing even more opportunities with other conditions.

As we continue to learn how ketamine works and watch the scientific evidence pile up, including our own clinical and anecdotal results, we envision ketamine will continue to revolutionize mental health. Plus, ketamine appears to have the ability to improve many other conditions and disease states because of its unique characteristics. For example, since ketamine has neural regenerative properties, we're seeing science show that it can be helpful with neurologic injury like stroke, and to the millions of people with mild to severe traumatic brain injury (TBI), as well as dementia.[18] This is due to the way ketamine fires up the BDNF to reverse brain atrophy. (There is even promising research showing ketamine can suppress proliferation of breast cancer cells.[19])

CHAPTER 6

THE KEY TO UNLOCK ANSWERS

I've been coping with depression and suicidal depression since before my college days, taking all kinds of depression and anti-anxiety medications among other things. When my 21-year-old son began battling suicidal depression, I realized I was mirroring him with my own feelings, and returning to a familiar mindset of not wanting to leave my bed in the mornings.

After reading about ketamine and how others felt creatively "unlocked" from the experience, I knew it was something I wanted to try.

In each of the three sessions, I had a different experience with something always waiting for me, helping unlock various parts of myself and my ability to be present. Now I'm more aware of my reactiveness to situations and I'm keen to explore those reactions—especially when I'm getting stressed out with my family, relatives, or friends. Now I try to slow down and step back to understand why I am getting upset, what I'm gaining from that feeling, and what impact that reaction might have. If that impact isn't worthwhile, how can it be different? Maybe a situation doesn't have to be stressful; maybe it can be more fun or at least viewed in a more positive way. It's like I'm finally compelled to reject the negative rather than running away from it.

I can also say "No" without having to make excuses. I recognize that everyone, including myself, is entitled to their emotions. I've also learned how to communicate more effectively with my husband, and to not make assumptions as to how he's feeling or his intentions. I feel like I'm able to listen to my family interact around me rather than getting involved or inserting myself when not necessary or warranted. And the kids, in particular, have noticed a difference.

Of course there's always an undercurrent of worry when my eldest son isn't doing so well. But now I am able to enjoy other parts of my life without feeling guilty, which is also new for me. I love and support my son, and, maybe most importantly, I am able to accept that he has his own reality to navigate and that's how it's supposed to be. My role is to be here for him and the rest of my family—in a happier and healthier headspace—should any of them want or need me.

—*Kristine, an actual patient of Field Trip*

Although we are highly recommending using ketamine to quickly improve your mental health, we are not suggesting that you buy it on the street and head to the club. Not only are street versions unsafe, but taking ketamine in an uncontrolled setting without medical supervision is a recipe for "bad trips" and possibly dangerous outcomes. As science continues to raise the potential for ketamine as a safe, powerful antidepressant, "ketamine clinics" have begun to pop up around the U.S. However, we have found several differences between the ketamine protocols described in this book and what is offered at other ketamine clinics. Plus, in this chapter, we're going to introduce ways ketamine can benefit couples, can be used in group settings, and can be particularly effective with war veterans.

First, and as noted above, we integrate the treatment with psychotherapy before, during, and after the *Exploration* sessions. We're seeking to leverage the power of a short-term psychedelic experience and applying psychotherapy for long-term behavioral change. Most ketamine clinics just treat ketamine as an antidepressant.

Second, we want to make sure people understand the difference between Ketamine-Assisted Psychotherapy and IV ketamine clinics and intranasal ketamine.

Ketamine infusion involves the client being infused with a continuous low dose of ketamine, requiring an intravenous insertion that is maintained throughout the session. Science shows that the positive effects from the ketamine infusion wear off within 24 to 48 hours, so the client needs to repeat the uncomfortable IV many times more than what we have seen necessary through the protocol described in this book. To achieve a longer-lasting benefit, IV clinics will "stack" the ketamine doses or repeat the procedure several times in a short amount of time. Research has found that stacking six doses of intravenous ketamine within a few weeks reduced the symptoms for only a month,[1] whereas our clients at Field Trip have improvements that are still present three months after their initial course of treatment. It is our hope that all IV ketamine clinics will add a mental health professional who can walk them through the protocol we describe in this book.

Intranasal ketamine applications, branded as Spravato, also seem to fade in days or in one to two weeks, which is why the patient takes the drug every one to two weeks indefinitely. This is because intranasal ketamine is a smaller, weaker form of ketamine compared to the potent, original form we use for Ketamine-Assisted Psychotherapy. Unlike Ketamine-Assisted Psychotherapy, which can often *replace* prescription antidepressants, intranasal Spravato is designed for people to stay on their existing medication.

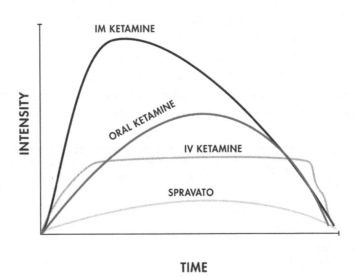

TIME

In either case—IV or intranasal—the results still don't last as long as most people would like. In the infusion model, clients often return every month. In the intranasal model, patients have to come back to the doctor's office every one to two weeks (since Spravato is administered only in doctors' offices). Also, when ketamine is used in these ways, it has only one target—depression.

IV ketamine clinics are often owned by physicians who are typically anesthesiologists with no training in mental health, and not psychiatrists. These doctors' offices are usually better suited for conventional Western approaches to medicine than whole-person-centered psychotherapy. Rarely do infusion centers and doctors' offices carry positive associations for most people. At larger IV ketamine clinics, nurses provide most of the care. Throughout the journey, they may pry your eyelids open to examine your pupils, which we don't do in Ketamine-Assisted Psychotherapy. In our opinion, these clinics address only the biological aspect of depression from a medical point of view. As we've stated, that's only half of the solution. When you add psychotherapy to this process, you gain specificity and can hypertarget the medicine to work on goals that are important to the client's life. Anecdotally, we often hear that the lack of psychological support through the journey and dosing at IV ketamine clinics is traumatizing for some.

Compared to IVs that deliver a steady state of ketamine intravenously over the course of about an hour, we suggest delivering all the medicine at the beginning of the *Exploration* session with a quick intramuscular (IM) shot, or oral ketamine in the form of a sublingual lozenge. We also advocate for dosing that considers the whole person, their experience, and the way they feel about the journey.

This is among other differences between ketamine and intranasal ketamine delivered in psychiatrists' offices or in IV ketamine clinics. Remarkably, the synergistic effects of combining the medicine with concurrent psychotherapy can more than *triple* the time needed before the next dose of the medicine (see below).

	IV Ketamine Clinics	Intranasal Ketamine (Spravato)	Ketamine-Assisted Psychotherapy
Typical frequency of stacking for severe depression	6 IV infusions of ketamine within 2–3 weeks	Twice per week for 4 weeks	6 Exploration sessions within 2–3 weeks
Psychotherapy (Preparation and Integration sessions)	No	No	Yes
Effects typically last	Approximately 1 month	Approximately 1 week	Approximately 3–4 months
Typical maintenance dosing	1 IV infusion per month	1 intranasal dose every 1–2 weeks	1 maintenance Exploration session every 2–12 months
Taken with concurrent prescription antidepressant	Not required	Required	Not required

If you do not live close to a Field Trip clinic, oral ketamine via Field Trip at Home™ is ideal for at-home applications. We also use it in-clinic for rare cases of needle phobia and under medical supervision for rare cases of extreme needle phobia. That being said, the needle we use is tiny and, unlike IV ketamine infusions, the "poke" lasts only a second.

Additionally, we suggest taking great care in creating a setting that nurtures a positive experience. Field Trip clinics, for example, feel like spas. Just this week as we were writing this chapter, we had a patient starting his ketamine journey. He walked through the door for the first time and said, "Wow! This looks like a resort!"

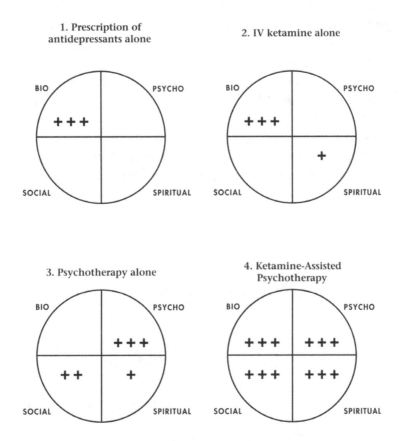

On average, people who complete our protocols experience significant improvements in depression and anxiety as measured by the nine-item Patient Health Questionnaire (PHQ-9) and the seven-item Generalized Anxiety Disorder scale (GAD-7), respectively. These gains are present three months after clients complete their initial course of treatment. That's about *three times longer* than the results coming out of IV ketamine studies. Some clients even report improvement lasting a year or more. When you combine psychotherapy with ketamine (the "other half of the equation" that IV clinics don't usually provide), you can also use it for a wider variety of concerns. We personally have found ketamine to be one of the most effective treatments for PTSD because while the ketamine immediately lifts the cloud of depression and stress, we can also help rewrite the memory from a new, perhaps more accurate, perspective during the *Exploration* session. When there are complex issues present like depression related to a person's autoimmune disease diagnosis, it's the medicine, the journey, and the psychotherapy together that change the way they think about themselves. Since ketamine usually brings trauma back to the surface, we typically start with lower doses in clients with PTSD as we slowly and safely reprocess traumatic memories.

These differences—how we administer ketamine, and how we approach the mindset, setting, and psychotherapy—yield a therapeutic dynamic that treats the biology, psychology, social, and spiritual areas of your life. This "whole person" approach gives the brain much more material to produce new neural pathways that result in positive behavioral change. (See diagram 4 on page 65).

Here is a sample KAP treatment plan for a client with treatment-resistant depression:

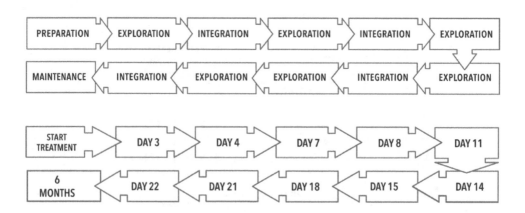

This example may or may not be right for you. We suggest approaching ketamine therapy in a highly personalized manner, so you may want more *Preparation* sessions, fewer *Exploration* sessions, and more *Integration* sessions. Your specific needs and related game plan will be discovered during the initial steps of the intake process.

One important decision will be about where and when you proceed with Ketamine-Assisted Psychotherapy. You can either visit one of the Field Trip clinics for an in-person journey, or we have developed a protocol for you to achieve your goals through an at-home experience. Let's take a look at that next.

CHAPTER 7

AT HOME: THE IDEAL MENTAL REBOOT

Not only was I overly conscious of how others perceived me, but I had a hard time speaking up for myself and vocalizing what I wanted. Being in a crowd, even during a standard Costco run, was enough to make my palms sweaty and send my mind into a panic.

For years I took selective serotonin reuptake inhibitors (SSRIs) and anti-anxiety medication. Four years ago, I lost my mother to cancer and the grief manifested into something I either couldn't or wouldn't let myself understand. She was not just my mother, but my rock. Though I was functioning, there was a huge void in my world that needed attention.

Although I'd done psychedelics recreationally when I was younger, they never led to mind-opening revelations. During the pandemic, I started digging into psychedelics further and that's when I discovered ketamine-assisted therapy and Field Trip.

From the sessions, I came to some life-changing realizations about myself, my thought patterns, and my coping mechanisms. It was also there that I learned I had been masking my own symptoms and that I had a compulsive need to make sure everyone around me was okay. The therapy allowed me to understand and manage my anxieties for the first time in years.

This entire experience has also changed my relationships. Now I seek connections with others by finding commonalities that will allow me to form more meaningful bonds. It's astounding to believe that such a low dose of ketamine could have such an earth-shattering and profound effect on my life. But it truly did. Through all of this I've decided to pursue what I'm passionate about, and now I am working toward goals.

—*Seth, an actual patient of Field Trip*

Not everyone can visit a licensed, medically supervised clinic like Field Trip. While Field Trip is in many major cities around the world, there are still many areas we don't serve. In fact, we suspect as Ketamine-Assisted Psychotherapy continues to be accepted as a legitimate, powerful therapeutic tool, that more and more people will seek the ideal mental vacation, and related breakthroughs, without leaving their home.

Considering the likelihood you may be reading this book and nowhere near one of our clinics, we wanted to outline a few recommendations so you can get the most from the experience at home. Remember that both in-clinic and at-home Ketamine-Assisted Psychotherapy require a prescription and are supervised by medical professionals. They can help you decide if at-home treatment via telemedicine is an option for you.

1. Overall, the protocol outlined throughout this book, with the intake, *Preparation*, *Exploration*, and *Integration* steps, will remain very similar with a few exceptions:

- While at home, you will connect with a licensed therapist, medical professional, or authorized adviser through an online video connection. Therefore, you'll need a computer or device with access to the Internet as well as a phone.

  Do not expect to fill out a quick form and have ketamine delivered within minutes. The intake procedure should include a highly personalized assessment, with honest discussions about any condition that may disqualify you from using ketamine. Just like in the clinic, you may be required to obtain a prescription via telemedicine with one of our medical providers while addressing the costs and related insurance coverages. This step is extremely critical for the overall experience to achieve the desired benefit.

- Refer to Chapter 9, "Ready to Board & Glossary," for details.

  After the intake process, you'll have a *Preparation* session with a licensed therapist, counselor, or coach via an online video meeting tool. Should you and the clinician agree that ketamine will be a good fit, and a treatment plan is prepared, a welcome package will be delivered to your home once you sign up for the program (which might include items like a copy of this book or another manual, a heart-rate monitoring device, perhaps some eyeshades, an access code to a related app (like the Field Trip app), and a suggested music playlist. The ketamine itself will typically be shipped directly from the compounding pharmacy to your house, so it may arrive in a separate package if it's not included in the welcome package.

- Read Part II of this book and complete the related sections for your mindset, intentions, and invocations.

2.   While preparing for your *Exploration* session, take care to identify the ideal setting for your experience. Choose a comfortable chair and a quiet room with low stimuli, calming colors, and low distractions. At the clinic, we created an ideal setting because we believe it's very important to facilitate the experience.

- Plan ahead so you have no visitors during this time, turn off your phone, and have the environment ready. Also, communicate in advance with your doctor, a close friend, or family member about your plans.

- We recommend having a journal or paper and pen nearby so when your session comes to an end, you can record what you saw, felt, and experienced.

3.   An *Integration* session should already be planned for the next day, if possible. This session can be conducted online or at a qualified therapist's office. Bring your journal or post-medicine notes (or drawings) along with your stated intentions. Your therapist will help interpret and analyze these materials to assist the therapeutic process.

Overall, your home can be a wonderful place to go deep inside your mind and make new discoveries. But we encourage you to be mindful of this medical procedure so that you're ready for the trip of your life.

CHAPTER 8

FREQUENTLY ASKED QUESTIONS

What is psychedelic medicine?

Psychedelic medicine refers to various techniques using psychedelic molecules for improving mental health and overall well-being. Scientifically, it is believed that the power of psychedelics to promote mental wellness and healing is the result of a temporary quieting of the ego and a suspension of the default mode network (DMN) of the brain. When combined with therapeutic support for integrating into your daily life, psychedelics can offer a path toward healing and transformation. Multiple evidence-based studies from world-class institutions have demonstrated that using psychedelics can produce profound, sustained results in as little as one session. Ongoing benefits include improved well-being and optimism, and increased neural plasticity.

Aren't psychedelics drugs of abuse? How is this different?

There is little evidence to suggest that experiences with psychedelic substances result in long-term addiction or physical harm, especially when taken in concert with psychotherapy. In fact, a growing set of studies indicates that these substances, when taken in a therapeutic setting, can be quite positive for mental health issues. They are paradoxically anti-addiction and help clients reduce or eliminate the use of alcohol or narcotics. However, as with any drug, there is potential for abuse and harm if not taken safely and under medical supervision. Field Trip promotes only the safe use of legal psychedelics under the supervision of our expert medical team in a therapeutic setting.

What about scary or "bad" trips?

Psychedelics are powerful substances that have the potential to cause profound changes in perception and patterns of thinking. They can be unpredictable and, at times, overwhelming for some people. With the *Preparation* session and the work you've done in this book, there is little risk of a "bad" trip. That said, often the challenging moments lead to the most significant breakthroughs and long-term benefits. Even difficult experiences can be wonderful opportunities to see life from a new perspective. Experienced professionals can help minimize the anxiety felt during the experience. They serve as trusted guides and interpreters while also maximizing the effectiveness of the treatment. By creating safe, comfortable environments and helping you establish an open, relaxed mindset, therapists help facilitate a beneficial experience.

Who are the providers?

At Field Trip, we use providers who are professionally trained and licensed medical practitioners. They are licensed physicians, nurse practitioners, and psychotherapists. Every Field Trip clinic has a medical director and mental health professionals on staff to screen our patients for safety and fit. All of our psychotherapists have been trained in using specific techniques and protocols during integration therapy. Field Trip also has a highly experienced and respected medical advisory team, made up of key opinion leaders in the mental health space, as well as scientific experts who have worked at major pharmaceutical organizations.

What conditions do you treat?

Currently, Field Trip has protocols for addressing depression and trauma, among many other conditions. (See Chapter 5: "Is Ketamine for You?") Program offerings may vary depending on the Field Trip center location since laws differ by country. Please reach out to us if you have questions about whether you qualify.

Are there conditions that would exclude me from treatment?

Although the use of ketamine therapy is generally safe for most individuals, there are some conditions that may disqualify you from this treatment. These conditions include, but are not limited to, pregnant women and nursing mothers, and individuals with a history of psychosis or schizophrenia, active mania/hypomania, or poorly controlled hypertension (high blood pressure) or hyperthyroidism.

Do note that high blood pressure that is well controlled with medication may not prevent you from benefiting from Ketamine-Assisted Psychotherapy. As a result, the medical team will assess blood pressure prior to ketamine administration. If your blood pressure is too high, unfortunately we will not be able to administer your medication, and your appointments will need to be rescheduled to ensure your safety. For details, see Chapter 5: "Is Ketamine for You?"

Do I need a referral?

In Canada, Field Trip currently requires a medical referral from your doctor or psychiatrist. If you are in Canada, you can download the referral form at fieldtriphealth.com. Once we have received a referral, our staff psychiatrist will screen prospective clients to ensure your safety and confirm KAP is the right fit for you.

In the U.S., Field Trip does not require a referral. To qualify for treatment, you will go through a secure medical intake questionnaire and conduct a consultation with one of our licensed medical professionals to ensure our program is the right fit.

How should I prepare? What can I expect?

During your consultation, our medical team will walk through the treatment process with you in detail. You will then be provided with additional resources and exercises to prepare for your initial ketamine experience. Our approach to KAP uses ketamine as a catalyst to unlock deeper therapy sessions with a trained psychotherapist. We then blend these intensive sessions with mindfulness, self-care, and personalized integration activities to deliver a holistic treatment approach that heals on multiple levels. See Chapter 6: "The Key to Unlock Answers."

How long is a treatment visit?

Our KAP protocol includes an initial medical consultation that is conducted virtually and takes approximately 45 minutes to one hour. After we determine that you are cleared for treatment and we find that the treatment is a good fit for you, we will schedule you in for your modules of *Preparation*, *Exploration*, and *Integration* sessions. The *Preparation* and *Integration* session(s) will take up to an hour each, while the *Exploration* sessions should be planned for two hours with an optional extra hour in our integration lounges for a total of up to three hours. The entire protocol is typically planned with your medical team and scheduled over a period of several weeks.

How many visits will I need to make?

Following your initial consultation, your therapeutic journey will be developed between you and your therapeutic team, but typically most people undergo four to six ketamine *Exploration* therapy sessions with four to six *Integration* therapy sessions. This will all take place over a period of approximately four weeks. After that initial phase, most people come back only periodically for a maintenance *Exploration* session experience to maintain the benefits they achieved through the initial program. Please note that the exact number of visits may vary by center location, by program, and by your response to the treatment.

Is this treatment covered under public health insurance in Canada?

As our psychedelic-assisted therapy program is still a novel treatment, our program is not currently covered under the Ontario Health Insurance Plan (OHIP) or other public health options in Canada.

Is this treatment covered by extended-benefit insurance providers?

As all sessions are conducted with licensed mental health professionals, you may be eligible for partial reimbursement under an out-of-network mental health benefit—the amount depending on your employer or insurer's coverage limits. In Ontario, this could be up to $2,225 of the total treatment cost. In the U.S., reimbursement amounts may vary depending on the insurance provider. Typically, only PPO (preferred provider organization) health insurance programs provide partial reimbursement for outpatient, out-of-network psychotherapy. You could receive up to $1,000 back directly for the total treatment costs.

We are happy to provide you with the necessary documentation to seek reimbursement from your insurance provider.

Is ketamine safe?

Yes. Ketamine-assisted therapy is conducted at lower doses of ketamine than what has been used safely in anesthesia for decades. It is known to be safe and well-tolerated in both healthy adults and children. Despite its common use in modern medicine, ketamine's application in lower dosages for the treatment of mental health challenges such as depression, anxiety, and PTSD is relatively new. During your consultation, our medical team will screen you carefully to ensure you are a safe candidate for our treatment.

How does ketamine work?

Ketamine is an NMDA receptor antagonist that interacts with many of your brain's neurotransmitters. Its effects can include relieving anxiety and pain, and acting as an antidepressant. Under medical supervision, lower doses of ketamine can relax your mind and allow you to temporarily disengage from your routine thought patterns. When combined with psychotherapy, studies have found that it can be helpful in reducing anxiety and depression. See Chapter 3: "How Ketamine Works Magic in the Brain."

How does ketamine feel?

Every psychedelic experience is unique to the individual and environment, and ketamine is no different. There are some commonalities in reported sensations from psychedelic doses of ketamine. You may experience a sense of disconnection—that you are observing your mind and body from outside rather than within. The experience has also been described as "euphoric," "calming," and "mystical." Many people experience changes in energy level, becoming either more relaxed or more energetic. The heart rate is often increased. It's important to recognize that for some people these unfamiliar sensations can be overwhelming or difficult. Even with experiences that may seem negative in the moment, the insights gained are often tremendously valuable.

Are there any side effects or risks?

As with any powerful substance, there are some potential side effects while under the influence of ketamine. Below are some potential effects you may experience during and after administration, until the effects of the drug have worn off:

- A feeling of dissociation or disconnection from your normal self
- A sense of impaired balance and coordination
- A feeling of drowsiness, mental confusion, and/or slurred speech
- Impacts to visual, auditory, or tactile processing, including diminished ability to see, hear, or feel objects accurately
- Worsening of psychotic symptoms in people who suffer from schizophrenia or severe personality disorder
- Feelings of anxiety, fright, nausea, and/or vomiting

More severe side effects are much more rare and typically seen only at much higher doses. These can include the following:

- Under surgical ketamine doses, there are reports of decreased immune function.

- Chronic, high-dose abuse of ketamine may cause urinary tract symptoms and permanent bladder dysfunction.

How is ketamine taken?

Ketamine can be administered to patients in a variety of ways, including intravenously, nasally, or sublingually (under the tongue). At Field Trip in Canada, patients consume tablets sublingually in the presence of a health professional. This means it typically takes effect within 5 to 10 minutes. Effects normally last from 45 to 75 minutes. In the U.S., Field Trip patients are given ketamine through an intramuscular injection, as opposed to "infusion" or IV clinics where the patient is connected intravenously throughout the session.

PART II

EXPERIENCING KETAMINE IN ACTION

CHAPTER 9

THE KAP WORKBOOK: READY TO BOARD & GLOSSARY

After offering our own personal experiences; explaining ketamine's revolutionary role in brain and psychotherapy; and ketamine's past, present, and future serving a wide range of conditions, you may be wondering, *How do I get started with ketamine?*

In some countries, you will need to have a medical referral from your primary care doctor or psychiatrist. In the U.S., a referral isn't necessary. To qualify for treatment, you will go through a secure medical intake questionnaire and conduct a consultation with a licensed medical professional to ensure ketamine is the right fit for you.

While the process may vary from practitioner to practitioner, the journey starts with the same essential steps:

- *Get in Touch.* There are a number of practitioners and clinics currently offering KAP, and the number is growing every day. The first step is to get in touch with them to determine whether you feel comfortable that the practitioner or clinic is well suited to help you on your journey.

- *Intake.* Any practitioner or clinic worth attending will conduct an intake with you to determine the appropriateness of KAP for your needs. You will be asked to complete a medical screening. This process will help the medical staff understand your situation. This initial conversation will cover your goals and identify any absolute contraindications that would suggest that you should not pursue KAP (see Chapter 1). If you're coming to a clinic with novel offerings like Field Trip, you can also decide whether to seek KAP for yourself, as a couple, or in a group setting. Additionally, you will decide whether you prefer to complete the KAP protocol from your home or in person with medical staff. You can start the intake process on the Field Trip website.

- *Insurance and Financial Concerns.* Some providers may ask you to pay for your first session in advance or provide a deposit to secure your first session. This is not uncommon. Payment plans and financing may also be available to support your therapy. As KAP is still a novel treatment, it is not generally covered by health insurance programs. We hope that will change in the years to come. However, you may be eligible for partial reimbursement under an out-of-network mental health benefit— the amount depending on your insurer's coverage limits. The provider should be able to give you a superbill to seek partial reimbursement directly from your health insurance company. You can call your health insurance company in advance to see whether it covers out-of-network mental health services, and to determine your deductible and the reimbursement rate.

- *Preparation Session.* Most providers will invite you to a *Preparation* session to have you meet your therapeutic team and prepare for your first session. This is typically conducted with a psychotherapist who will be guiding you through your ketamine journey. During this session, you and your therapist will determine a recommended treatment plan, including the number of *Exploration* and *Integration* sessions you may need.

For example, we suggest clients with severe treatment-resistant depression complete six *Exploration* sessions within two to three weeks or so (see diagram on page 64. The "stacking" of *Exploration* sessions in a short amount of time has been shown to be effective for this condition; and "stacking" them close together is less important in other conditions. This plan will include a *Preparation* session, and then *Integration* sessions that follow the first, second, fourth, and sixth *Exploration* sessions. Someone with mild anxiety or depression may need only two *Exploration* sessions and two *Integration* sessions. However, someone with untreated PTSD may need more *Exploration* sessions—since we typically want to start with lower doses of ketamine and gradually increase the dose when trauma is present. As you can see, this protocol is highly personalized. Regardless of the number of sessions, we suggest using a journal prior to and after each *Exploration* session, giving your therapist insight to further the healing process. Your response to treatment as it unfolds can help you and your provider make a decision on how many *Exploration* sessions you will need.

We encourage you to discuss your plans with any health-care professionals you're working with, from your primary care physician to your psychotherapist and/or psychiatrist. This will help them understand the positive changes that are imminent in your life, and feel more free to recommend KAP to others. When speaking with your doctor—and family for that matter—assure them you are undergoing a treatment that is safe, proven to be effective, and administered by licensed health-care professionals. You can use the material in this book to help answer any of their questions.

HOW TO USE THE FOLLOWING GUIDE

We're going to walk you through three types of sessions. Chapter 10 will walk you through *Preparation* sessions, Chapter 11 will walk you through *Exploration* sessions, and Chapter 12 will walk you through *Integration* sessions.

We have included a series of tools, journal entry guides, sample invocations, and worksheets to facilitate your own personalized experience.

We believe this will become a wonderful resource to record your growth. As you step inside and dig deep, it's our hope that you find your truest self. Enjoy the journey.

GLOSSARY: NEW TERMINOLOGY FOR YOUR JOURNEY

Before we dive into the ketamine protocol, we suggest becoming familiar with the following vocabulary and meaning for the experiences. Psychedelic therapists and psychedelic researchers tend to use a common lexicon to talk about these experiences. As a client, it's helpful to have a basic understanding of these terms, listed in alphabetical order.

Afterglow. *Afterglow* is a term often used to describe the positive physical and mental effects that can last from a couple of days to a couple of weeks following a psychedelic experience. This state of "glow" is characterized by feelings of increased psychological clarity, inner peace, or states of awe and bliss.

Psychiatrist Walter Pahnke describes afterglow as an "elevated and energetic mood with a relative freedom from concerns of the past and from guilt and anxiety."

While the psychedelic medicine still lingers within the body and mind, be sure to create intentional time and space to reflect on your journey while in this expansive state. This introspection can include journaling, creating art, listening to the same music you experienced during your journey, or moving your body through dance, exercise, or yoga. We will give you several suggestions in the section on *Integration* sessions.

Ceremony. The word *ceremony* is used to describe any activity performed with a sense of sacredness and formality. In many Indigenous cultures, psychedelic plants are considered sacred—purely ceremonial, never recreational. Under the guidance and supervision of a shaman or the spiritual leader of the community, any compounds would be administered for very clear reasons, such as for an initiation rite or healing ceremony. A ceremony can begin days or weeks before your dosing and may involve avoiding intoxicants like alcohol and other drugs; eliminating certain things from your diet, like sugar, salt, or spices; and changing your lifestyle by avoiding normal sexual activity or consuming media.

A ceremony may also encompass a practice or ritual that marks the beginning and/or continues throughout your experience, often with the intention to pay homage and extend gratitude to the medicine and the sacred wisdom it comes from. There are ways to create a ceremony at home for yourself by reflecting upon what's important to you. We'll help you get very specific about your intention in the *Preparation* session section that follows. Perhaps your intention is very specific, or maybe you're open to whatever unfolds. Perhaps there's an album/soundtrack or a symbol that you want to bring with you on your journey. Creating our own rituals before, during, or after a journey is an opportunity to approach them with a purpose and presence, bringing our full selves to the experience and what it's meant to teach us, and remembering the shoulders we stand upon when working with these medicines.

Container. A container is a metaphorical reference to the safe physical and sensory holding space in which true transformation and healing can take place.

The container may consist of the physical setting, the connection among the group, the words shared, and/or the rituals and practices that take place. Healing can be beautiful on its own, but the act of getting there—especially through the psychedelic experience—can initiate sensitive or challenging memories and moments. A safe container enables and empowers support during this process.

Decriminalize. To decriminalize is to remove or reduce the criminal legal classification or status of a particular substance or action associated with the substance. While ketamine is legal and FDA-approved as an analgesic and for treatment-resistant depression, efforts are being made to decriminalize psilocybin and MDMA, among other compounds classified as psychedelics. Decriminalization of psychedelic medicines is a step in the right direction, as we believe no one should be penalized for using medicines that improve the quality of their lives.

DMN (Default Mode Network). See Chapter 3 for more information. The DMN is a system in the brain that orients us to who we think and believe we are—our ego—and how we relate to the world around us, particularly at rest. The DMN is active when we are not focused on the outside world, and instead are preoccupied with internal mind-wandering or daydreaming. Ketamine, like other psychedelics, temporarily disables the DMN, giving us a perspective without our own ego attached.

Drop In. "Dropping In" is slang that describes the process of easing into a consciousness-altered state. Oftentimes, people will turn off their phones, get in a comfortable position, and prepare themselves to drop in to their journey.

Ego Death (aka Ego Dissolution). During a journey, the DMN, the area of the brain known to be responsible for our ego, has been shown to be quieted. This contributes to the experience known as ego death or ego dissolution. This is why people often speak of returning from trips with a renewed perspective on themselves and the world. Prior to a true ego dissolution during a psychedelic treatment, the ego identity shapes the perception of what we know of as the Self. The quieting, or even fully dissolving, of the ego allows for a new perspective of ourselves, our world, and our place in it.

Psychedelics are a powerful way to help us get out of our own way, so to speak, to detach from the shade of our ego and confront the protective walls it has built.

Entheogen. Entheogens are plant-derived psychedelic medicines that produce a non-ordinary state of consciousness. These altered states can include shifts in perception, mood, consciousness, cognition, or behavior. Often, entheogens complement practices aimed toward achieving transcendence, like meditation, yoga, prayer, trance, chanting, ecstatic dance, and more. Entheogenic plants and fungi include peyote and San Pedro cacti; the vine and shrub used to make ayahuasca; psilocybin mushrooms; and the root bark of the iboga shrub. Entheogens have been used for millennia for healing, knowledge, creativity, and spiritual connection. Over the last decade, scientific research has also demonstrated that these plants and fungi can treat a range of chronic illnesses, such as depression, and conditions such as grief that can be especially challenging to break through.

Healer. Similar to a guide and shaman, a healer uses sacred and spiritual modalities to transfer energy through themselves to a recipient. These modalities promote self-healing by relaxing the body, releasing tensions, and strengthening the body's own immune system. Healers have the intention of bringing the recipient into a state of balance and well-being on all levels.

Heroic Dose. Heroic dose or transformational dose refers to a relatively large dose of psychedelic medicine being administered. Before experiencing a heroic dose, we recommend discussing your intentions, experience with psychedelics, and purpose for therapy. Typically, we will offer incremental doses until we reach the state recommended from the therapist or doctor. This "low and slow" approach gives you the opportunity to discern how you're reacting to these experiences on both an emotional and psychological level. *Heroic dose* is usually a term people use when talking about classical psychedelics like psilocybin. In Ketamine-Assisted Psychotherapy, a heroic dose may be akin to what we typically refer to as a high-dose session.

Holding Space. *Holding space* is a term often used in psychedelic therapy, but it can extend to any human interaction with the intent to drop in together. Holding space for another person involves being completely present and inviting whatever is coming up for them in that moment to be shared and bared. In this safe space, what is released is not judged, questioned, or interfered with. It is simply heard, seen, and received.

In group settings, holding space becomes increasingly important in order to find cohesion among the different states and perspectives of all individuals in the group. A guide or facilitator's role is to hold space for their client or group during intention-setting/integration circles as well as during the trip itself.

Integration. During and after an *Exploration* session with ketamine, you may have profoundly new or altered insights or awareness about yourself, your life, and your emotions. You will also experience a period of neuroplasticity, during which the brain's ability to form and reorganize pathways and connections is increased. But to help these realizations become lasting change, and to make the most of your more neuroplastic brain, it's important to integrate your new insights and perspectives with a therapist. Traditionally, integration means "bringing parts together to make whole," so by blending the learnings from your journey into different areas of your life, you can turn your insights into a tangible and comprehensive reality. Integration can include physical, somatic, psycho-spiritual, and emotional work to bring your journey into your lived reality. For example, if you've experienced trauma with someone in your life that you couldn't shake previously, but your trip enabled you to see the memory with a new lens, then integration work could involve reflection, journaling, forgiveness practices, working with a therapist, or even movement and music.

Intention(s). An intention is a goal, a vision, an aim, and a purpose for your journey and therapy. When working with the medicine, setting intentions prior to your journey will ground you and shed light on how the experience could heal or benefit you. It's a critically important part of the process.

Landing. Once the high of the psychedelic medicine begins to taper off, there's a period of coming down, sometimes referred to as landing, comedown, or reentry. As your state of consciousness returns to normal, you may experience myriad physical and emotional effects depending on the experience you've just had. For example, if you've had an uncomfortable or anxious experience, the landing may feel relatively pleasant as you ground yourself in the present moment again, as Ronan described in his journey at the beginning of the book. Alternatively, if you've had an epic trip, landing may feel a little disappointing, because it's a return to "reality." This landing phase usually happens gradually and may last up to 24 hours or more, depending on which psychedelic you've taken, how much, and even how frequently you've experienced a similar kind of trip. During this time, it's recommended that you rest and drink plenty of non-caffeinated fluids, as well as notice any physical responses, just in case you may need to reach out to someone for additional support. It may take some time to feel like you're fully back in your physical body, which is why grounding experiences like yoga can be helpful.

Legalize. Unlike decriminalization, legalization of psychedelics is a legal regime in which production, distribution, and possession of psychedelics is expressly authorized by the government, subject to certain regulations. While we believe decriminalization is a positive, we believe the biggest impact of psychedelic therapies will be achieved through legalization.

Mantra. An ancient practice in which a word or sound is repeated to aid concentration in meditation. This could be a phrase that embodies your intention—like "I belong" or "everything is as it should be." Mantras originated thousands of years ago and are traditionally spoken in Sanskrit, the most common being "om." In the next section, we'll help you find a type of mantra that can help you in your *Exploration* session.

Meditation. The practice of deep breathing, mindfulness, and/or guided visualization that either nurtures a state of complete and total presence or transcendence. When you achieve presence or transcendence, neither the past nor the future exist. A deep meditative state is the essence of just *being*. This practice is a powerful tool to find calm and inner peace while enhancing awakening to what is and what shall be.

Mystical. Psychedelics offer access to your personal subconscious—the space where unresolved grief, guilt, trauma, and more usually live—as well as an opportunity to connect to a collective consciousness where mystical experiences can happen. This collective consciousness is usually perceived as a greater force, which many call the universe, God, Source, etc. For thousands of years, ancient mystics, sages, and saints have described experiences with this greater energy. The core characteristic of a mystical experience is a sense of connectedness that in our modern-day lives can feel deeply gratifying. When we feel disconnected, our nervous systems are in fight-or-flight mode, which can create many emotional and physical repercussions over the long haul, and stress is often at the root of many illnesses. The parasympathetic nervous system, on the other hand, is where rest, relaxation, and repair can happen. Additional elements of the mystical experience include feeling a sense of oneness and unity, transcending time and space, a sacred experience where words aren't enough to define what you've gone through, becoming aware of an ultimate reality, and a deep sense of positivity. We often use the Mystical Experience Questionnaire designed to measure your subjective experience of mystical experiences in a session since they tend to be correlated with mood improvement.

Oneness. Would you believe that *Forbes* reported that a sense of oneness may be the key to happiness? A study published in the journal *Psychology of Religion and Spirituality* revealed that no matter what religion a person identifies with, a feeling of oneness is linked to greater satisfaction in life. But what, exactly, is oneness? Oneness can be described as the sense that everything in the world is interdependent and influenced by each other. Oneness can also be experienced as related to social connectedness, connectedness to nature, empathy for others, and life satisfaction. If you feel that sense of oneness, it can be a core part of your makeup, rather than a fleeting state, so it's not dependent upon a mood or a situation but rather a general attitude toward life. Psychedelic experiences can often activate this sense of oneness by dissolving the ego. Ketamine-Assisted Psychotherapy can help you move from merely understanding a theory about oneness to having an actual experience in which "all is one."

Outcomes. Outcomes are a zoomed-out view of how your embodied intentions resulted from the psychedelic experience. How did your trip turn out compared to this scenario? How do you feel about what was or wasn't in alignment with your vision? What lessons can you take into your day? What new lessons or growths occurred as a result? Outcomes may also be used in a more clinical, objective way (e.g., assessing improvement in depressive symptoms).

Prayer/Invocations. A series of words or phrases written or spoken to help you center or invoke or channel your highest or wisest self, or if you're religious or spiritual, a higher power. Prayer/invocations could apply to anyone of all religious or spiritual backgrounds as the intention is the same: to connect with something bigger than yourself. We'll help you select an invocation in the next section.

Psychedelic. The word *psychedelic* is a combination of two Greek words: *psyche* (meaning "mind" or "soul") and *delos* (meaning "unconcealed" or "manifested"). It was used in the 1950s by Humphry Osmond, a British psychiatrist working in Canada at the time. "To fathom hell or soar angelic / Just take a pinch of psychedelic," he wrote in a letter to Aldous Huxley. Huxley, one of the most well-known names in psychedelics, went on to write *The Doors of Perception* and change the course of history for psychedelic interpretation.

Psychonaut. One who frequently explores altered states of consciousness.

Rebirth or Renewal. On the heels of an ego death experience follows a period of rebirth, or awakening. By shedding who we think we are (based on our past, material possessions, beliefs, and judgments), we uncover who we truly are at our core. This is the process of awakening that puts us in a position to let go of or heal past wounds and traumas.

Release. Release comes before renewal. To release is to identify and let go of things that no longer serve you.

Set and Setting. There are two elements that should not be overlooked before and during a journey. Together, they refer to the conditions under which the journey is taken. *Set* refers to the internal conditions: the person's mental and emotional states, personality, beliefs, and intentions. *Setting* refers to physical space and the surrounding environment in which the journey takes place: the location, noises, sights, decor, music, and any people who might be with you during the journey. Though the ideal setting will vary from person to person (some individuals like to be alone, while others prefer social settings), a supportive and shame-free environment is always essential.

Shadow (Carl Jung Definition). In storytelling, shadows are often depicted as menacing, dark, lurking, and creepy. There's a reason for that. Swiss psychologist Carl Jung believed that to become enlightened, we must first learn to accept the parts of ourselves that our ego doesn't want to accept. The more we suppress our shadows, the denser and darker they become. But on the flip side, when we acknowledge and integrate those difficult-to-embrace aspects of ourselves, we strip our shadows of the power they have on our unconscious thoughts, emotions, and behaviors. In Jungian terms, the *shadow* or *shadow self* is a part, or parts, of us that we may deny, hide, and reject. Maybe this happened for good reason, when it was a survival or adaptive technique to make it through a tough period of our lives. Maybe it occurred for us to fit in with the morals we learned from our family, communities, and society. Maybe it happened for reasons we've long forgotten. Psychedelics can surface what's in our subconscious or our shadow. When we don't acknowledge these repressed aspects of our unconscious self, they can control us and impact how we think, feel, and engage with the world around us. According to Jung, "Until you make the unconscious conscious, it will direct your life and you will call it fate."

Shaman. In Indigenous cultures throughout South America and Asia, a shaman is a person believed to have an open connection to the spirit world. In other words, they're believed to be more lucid to what isn't part of our physical reality. Many shamans have a deep understanding of psychedelics and their healing properties, especially since their experience with psychedelics are purely medicinal, never recreational. Shamans aren't limited to purely ancient tribal roles; they exist today. Many modern-day shamans can assist in people's healing journeys with psychedelics. Be mindful of who you work with. Given the popularity of plant medicine and even plant medicine tourism, do your research on the person you choose to work with to ensure that they will guide you with clear intention and real experience.

Somatic. The term *somatic* relates to the body, and very often people will pair psychedelic therapies with different forms of somatic body work. As we hold traumas and stresses in our bodies in different ways, psychosomatic conditions refer to physical symptoms that result from psychological triggers or ailments.

Surrender. Psychedelics are "nonspecific amplifiers," which is a scientific way of saying that they intensify whatever feelings the person is already experiencing, whether those feelings are "good" or "bad" (hence the word *nonspecific*). It's through this amplification that we start to see more clearly. The practice of surrendering, in the context of a psychedelic experience, often means releasing resistance to whatever is coming through for you: good and bad. The ability to surrender is also deeply connected to the environment where the experience is taking place (the setting). When you're in a supportive environment, you are more likely to surrender and be present to the messages that you are becoming aware of throughout the journey.

Synesthesia. *Synesthesia* describes the experience of a convergence of our senses: feeling something that they see, tasting something that they hear, and so forth. For instance, many people who have psychedelic experiences report "seeing" music or that certain words or numbers are associated with certain colors. Artists and authors such as Edgar Allan Poe and Samuel Taylor Coleridge are reported to have been inspired by psychedelic-induced synesthesia. Functional magnetic resonance imaging studies of people during psychedelic experiences demonstrate that different parts of the brain light up during a journey, which may explain the synesthesia that occurs during a trip.

Tripping. To be in an altered state of consciousness.

TLO (Trust, Let Go, Be Open). A mantra used by psychedelic therapists and practitioners coined at the Johns Hopkins Center for Psychedelic and Consciousness Research.

Turn On, Tune In, Drop Out. American psychologist Timothy Leary popularized the phrase "Turn on, tune in, drop out" to describe the phases that make up the psychedelic experience. In the words of Leary himself, to turn on means to "activate your neural and genetic equipment." It's the act of becoming lucid to the idea that there's more to the universe than what our physical senses can comprehend in the day-to-day. Psychedelic medicine is often the catalyst for this first step of turning on. The next step, tuning in, means to take your new inner awareness and apply it to your interactions with the external world, whether that be nature, other people, or physical materials. Lastly, to drop out means to lovingly disengage with that which isn't serving you anymore. Although Leary is often criticized for some of his reviews, including people misinterpreting the intention of this statement to justify leaving society altogether, we believe that there is much merit to his commentary here; that psychedelic journeys empower you to become increasingly aware of who you are and what you want, and empower you to let go of those things that don't matter. It's no different than the adage "Don't sweat the small stuff . . . and it's all small stuff."

CHAPTER 10

THE KAP WORKBOOK: THE PREPARATION SESSION

This chapter is your guide to your *Preparation* session, which takes place a day or two before your first *Exploration* session. During your *Preparation* session, you will meet with your therapist to prepare for the journey ahead. The goals of the *Preparation* session are twofold. The first is to set an intention for the journey that lies ahead of you. The second is to become familiar with every step of the KAP protocol. This tends to enhance the effects of the medicine, puts your mind at ease, and helps you get excited for your journey.

Complete the activities in this section *before* meeting with your therapist for your *Preparation* session. Discuss any insights, goals, and concerns, as everything you bring to this work will enhance the journey ahead of you. You will refer back to several of these activities throughout your journey, so be sure to bring this book to all of your sessions.

This chapter includes the following activities:

1. Listen to the Preparation Meditation

2. Write Your Personal Mantra

3. Set Your Intention and Select Invocation

4. Consider Special Objects

5. Read "What to Expect"

6. Prepare Mind, Body, and Spirit for the Journey

7. Read "The Guest House" by Rumi

1. Listen to the Preparation Meditation

You can read all the research we've introduced you to in Part I of this book, but an objective understanding of *what* is happening in your brain is quite different from *how* altered states feel subjectively. To give you a preview of how these states feel, the first activity in this chapter is reading and listening to the preparation meditation below. This meditation includes clinical hypnosis, which, like ketamine sessions, is considered a non-ordinary state of consciousness. In fact, brain scans have shown that both hypnosis and ketamine suspend the brain's default mode network (DMN), which you learned about in Chapter 3. Many people describe both hypnosis and ketamine-induced states as being suspended somewhere in between being asleep and being awake. Others say it's like dreaming. Listening to this meditation is particularly helpful for clients who have no previous experience with ketamine or other psychedelic medicines. You can listen to this track in the Field Trip app, which can be downloaded onto your phone.

Consider this meditation your training wheels. In terms of intensity, the preparation meditation is usually around a 2 or 3 on a scale of 1 to 10—depending on how hypnotizable you are and how much experience you have with meditation, guided imagery, and hypnosis. During your *Exploration* session, the medicine will take the intensity up to about a 7 or 8 on a scale of 1 to 10—depending on your dose. In this moment, notice how that makes you feel. Are you excited about the journey ahead? Nervous? Hopeful? Remember that KAP is a highly personalized approach. The way you feel during this phase can help us determine your dose when it comes time for your *Exploration* session.

This preparation meditation can teach you how to relax into a deep state of trance. When you do so, you'll have an actual experience of what it feels like when the brain's DMN is turned down. Remember, the DMN is the "me, me, me" network associated with our ego. Using this meditation can dissolve some of the apprehension when you experience the ego going offline. It can also be helpful to use this practice as a rehearsal for the *Exploration* session. Listen to this track with an eye mask on and comfortably reclined or lying down, just like you'll be doing when you receive the ketamine. Get used to the experience of darkness, since the medicine usually makes the physical world fade to black before any colorful visuals emerge.

Unless you have experience with psychedelic medicine, the actual subjective experience is unique. Some clients notice a few seconds of clinging or confusion when ordinary consciousness fades away during an *Exploration* session. Breathe into it. Tell the ego: *You'll be back. This is only temporary. It's okay to let go.* After all, most depressive and anxious thoughts are rooted in the ego—since they are concerned with *I* or *me* (e.g., *What if I'm not okay? Is something wrong with me?*). We often forget how connected we are to others. Having an experience where you have an inner sense that "all is one" is a potent antidote to these negative thoughts and feelings.

Many people enjoy the way the medicine feels. It can initially make you feel a little floaty—similar to the way laughing gas feels. Anecdotally, most people with experience with psychedelics say the colors of a ketamine journey are darker (e.g., black, rich purples, dark blues) compared to other psychedelics. Others may have a moment of apprehension when they sense themselves crossing the bridge that separates this ordinary world from the "special world" of a ketamine journey, which usually occurs within 1 to 3 minutes with an intramuscular ketamine injection or within 15 minutes with ketamine taken orally.

It's like the moment you board a roller coaster. Some people are more excited, while others are a bit nervous. Just greet the way you're feeling with awareness. Hold the feeling without judgment, because there is no right or wrong way to feel. You can also take comfort in knowing that we use the way you feel to determine your starting dose. When using this meditation, it can be helpful to remember the phrase you'll hear in it:

Trust, Relax, and Let Go.

This simple mantra tends to be very helpful during the *Exploration* session, so use the preparation meditation as a time to practice saying this to yourself. After you read the meditation (or listen to the recording on the Field Trip app) one or more times, we'll have you write a short, personal mantra that you can say silently to yourself after you take the medicine.

Here is the script for the preparation meditation.

PREPARATION MEDITATION

This is a meditation to prepare you for psychedelic-assisted therapy. And many people say that this practice can even mimic psychedelics and know how it may feel for you . . . which, of course, can ease your mind and relieve any anxiety you may have about the experience.

So let's begin this journey today by simply noticing the way the body is already beginning to settle in and relax. The hands can find a comfortable place to rest . . . just there, that's right. As you prepare yourself for this meditation, any tension around the forehead, the eyes, and the neck can release. . . . And then, when you're ready to really let go, you can close your eyes. And now just allowing relaxation to unfold at its own pace . . . taking all of it as it comes . . .

You're listening to my voice . . .
You're breathing in and out . . .
And you're becoming more and more relaxed . . .
The body feels cool, calm, and comfortable.
The breath moves naturally . . .
And perhaps you notice the place in the mind or body where you already feel a bit of a light trance.
That's right, that's right . . .
And once you notice that relaxation, you can allow the trancelike state to grow . . .

Isn't it interesting how altered states of consciousness can unfold in this natural way. After all, you've probably already experienced light forms of altered states . . . when you go somewhere else in your mind . . . or meditate . . . or experience awe and connection when watching the sun rise . . . or have been mesmerized by music or flashing lights or a drum circle . . . or experienced the floaty feeling that comes with laughing gas or anesthesia . . . And in this practice today, you may be reminded of one of those experiences . . . As you recall the memory in this way, a feeling of them may begin to unfold . . .

And this relaxation will probably begin to unfold . . . in its own natural way . . . and you can simply take it as it comes . . . and I wonder if you can also cultivate a gentle, open, and curious attitude as you go deeper. Many people say this gentle curiosity helps them to have positive experiences with psychedelics. That open and curious attitude can help you through your journey, and if you see a door, you can walk through it . . . If you see a window, you can open it . . . If you see a stairway, you can climb it . . . and experience any physical sensations or feelings. If there is a moment of apprehension, you can move toward the experience instead of running away from it. And many people say this experience is a metaphor for what is happening in their lives. Whatever you find in your journey, it can be easy to trust, relax, and let go . . .

When you're ready to go deeper, you can become even more still by noticing the sounds you hear . . . beginning with the loudest sound you hear . . . and I wonder if you can hear with your entire being . . . and now, moving to a medium sound . . . and when you're ready to become even more still . . . notice the quietest sound you can hear at this moment.

And now, moving to your sense of sight. . . . Isn't it interesting that even with the eyes closed, there are so many colors on the back of the eyelids? Notice one in front of you. . . . And now, on the next inhale, roll the eyeballs all the way and hold the breath and hold the eyeballs up. . . . And now exhaling and allowing the eyeballs to float down, down, down. . . . That's right.

Now you see a garden . . . and in that garden is a stairway. . . . In your mind's eye, you can see yourself walking to the top of that stairway now . . . and you look down, and you see the most magical place you've ever seen . . . a place that some part of you knows will help you cultivate peace in a way that may be so deep that it feels spiritual . . . or, perhaps, connecting with power that may, for some, feel that it's connecting to some universal source or being.

Walking down this stairway now . . .

Stepping down the stairway with the right foot, stepping down with the left foot . . .

Feeling the body descend, hearing the foot making contact with the stair as you go even deeper now, deeper and deeper, more and more. . . . And you can allow yourself to go into this dreamy state, a state that can feel like you're some-where in between being awake and being asleep. . . . And it can feel so relaxing . . . so calming. . . . That's right, and the body feels even more relaxed and the mind, too, is so calm . . . that's right. That's right. Deeper and deeper, more and more. Trust, relax, let go. Trust, relax, let go.

And now, or at some point in this practice today, it's natural to notice how the ego—the part of you that knows you are you—has probably already begun to soften or will at some point of your journey today. . . . Send a message to your ego now: Tell it, "You'll be back." In psychedelic journeys, you may feel the ego trying to tightly grip on as the medicine begins to work. . . . The more you loosen the grip, the more peaceful journeys tend to be. If it feels like the ego is dying, tell it, "You're okay. You'll be back soon." . . . Trust, relax, and let go.

It can be helpful to mindfully become aware of that part of you, . . . so in your mind's eye, you see the part of you that knows you are you . . . the part of you that you refer to as "I" or "me." Your name . . . where you live . . . what you do, . . . and, also, a sense of the body and space and time . . . how tall you are . . . your age relative to time . . . a sense of the body sitting here, which is typically experienced as being separate from others . . . and with this sense of self come thoughts and feelings . . . all the things you need to do. . . . And in your mind's eye, you have a sense of this that you call "I" or "me."

And as I count up from 1 to 7 . . . you can imagine that all these things—ego, body, space, and time—turning into gold dust that's being blown away . . .

1 . . . 2 . . . 3 . . . 4 . . . 5 . . . 6 . . . 7

Now, I wonder if you can notice the immersion of pure being . . . of pure awareness. . . . Many people say that this helps them to feel an experience of one-ness in relation to an inner world within. . . . Others say this feels like a fusion of your personal self into a larger whole. . . . Others feel awe and connection . . . or, perhaps, even sacred. And if you have even a small sense of any of these feelings, then you already know what psychedelic medicine is likely to make you feel. . . . Isn't that so nice to know?

I'm not sure what this pure being will help you to do. Or are you feeling joy or peace? Or perhaps, a feeling of peace and tranquility? In this pure awareness, you can simply enjoy this experience . . . nothing to bother, nothing to do. That's right. Many people say this gives them perspective once they emerge back into their waking life. . . .

Now, as I count backward from 5 to 1, you will be presented with some sort of insight. It may be something small, like *This feels nice; I really need more of this pure awareness to recharge in my life.* For others, it can be a profound insight, like the true roots of any struggles you're experiencing. For others, it can feel like a sense of universal love that is the antidote to your worldly experience.

5 . . . 4 . . . 3 . . . 2 . . . 1 . . . You can hear and feel that insight, can't you?

And now remember what you got from this journey today . . . and lean into your next journey of a non-ordinary state of consciousness with excitement . . . curiosity . . . openness . . . for you.

Come back to this garden of pure awareness often . . .

Whether it's with this track or with psychedelic-assisted therapy.

And now, see the stairway that brought you here.

Consciousness will return to the body.

You'll become more awake and alert as you walk up the stairs now.

1 walking up

2 with a sense of power now

3 taking with you a sense of this inherent peace

4 feeling so rejuvenated, so restored

5 feeling the body move up now as consciousness returns fully to the body

6 halfway up now

7 taking a big step up into feeling so awake, so alive

8 giving a little wiggle to your fingers and your toes

9 up and awake

10 awake and alive

11 so reinvigorated

12 eyes open, awake, alive

2. Write Your Personal Mantra

Your personal mantra is simply a phrase that's one to five words you can say silently to yourself when you're crossing the bridge from the ordinary world to the special world of the ketamine journey. You can also use your personal mantra if you encounter a moment of confusion or apprehension in the journey. There were a few phrases you read or heard in this meditation:

Let go . . .

Gentle, curious, and open . . .

Trust, relax, and let go . . .

Some other examples include variations of these phrases or even simple, one-word mantras:

Breathe.

Trust.

I'm okay.

Leap.

I'm safe.

Open the heart.

It's okay to let go.

Go deeper.

Let go.

Let it be easy. (Ronan's personal mantra.)

What do you know about yourself? Are you an open, fearless, extroverted explorer who has previous experience with psychedelic medicine? If so, perhaps your mantra will be *Go deeper.* Or, are you someone who struggles with giving up control who has never used psychedelics? If so, perhaps the appropriate mantra for you is *Let go.* Is there anxiety or trauma that lives in the body? If so, perhaps *Breathe* feels right. Do any of these words or phrases resonate with you? If not, write your own personal mantra. Remember that it should be no longer than five words, because ketamine will temporarily disable the complex thinker within you.

My own personal mantra is _____

_____ .

Remind yourself of this personal mantra during your *Exploration* session. It can be a very helpful phrase as your journey with the medicine begins.

3. Set Your Intention and Select Invocation

Why were you called to do this deep work? What is it that you need? What would you like to shift or change in your life? Your intention may shift or pivot through this process, so you may want to come back to this page as your journey unfolds to see if your original intention still fits.

Answer this question with an open heart and mind. Get vulnerable. Don't intellectualize or use the complex thinker in you. In fact, the very first answer that comes up tends to be the one that is rising up from the inner healing intelligence within you. For some, this intention may even be just one word. Intentions tend to be short and guide the longer, poetic invocation you can write for yourself. Most of the *Preparation* session with your therapist is devoted to discussing and making sense of your intention.

Some examples of intentions we've used include "Let my light shine brighter," "See my self-worth," "Bring your voice back," and "Be fully present instead of having one foot out the door."

My intention for this journey is _____

_____ .

Now that you have your intention, it's time to prepare your invocation. There are three options for invocations:

1. Write your own invocation.

2. Select an invocation.

3. Ask that your therapist write an invocation for you.

We find that clients who take the time to write their own invocation report profoundly powerful, healing, and intentional journeys. Provide this written invocation to your therapist to read to you just as you are taking the medicine during your first *Exploration* session. Some people stay with the same invocation throughout several *Exploration* sessions. Others find that the intention organically changes as they move through *Exploration* and *Integration* sessions.

Having your invocations written down in this book can be quite helpful. Should you return for a *Maintenance* session, you may want to go back to your original intention and invocation or, if you'd like, write a new one. When the words of your invocation are the last words you hear or read before you begin your ketamine journey, it primes your mind, body, and spirit to cross the threshold into the therapeutic experience. It can add a great deal of specificity and intention to the journey.

To determine whether you want to write your own invocation, select one, or have one written for you, read the sample invocations included below and see if any of them speak to you. Remember: You can stay with one invocation through all of your *Exploration* sessions. Or, you can change your invocation as you move through this journey.

Sample Invocations

Here's an example of an invocation from a client I worked with. As you can see, her intention was to realize her full self and become free. The poetic intention of her words served as a wonderful way to trust, relax, and let go into the ketamine journey. As is often the case, the images, sensations, and worlds she saw were guided by the words she wrote.

It's safe for the chains to come off.
It's safe to be who you are.
It's safe when people don't like you.
It's safe to come out of the cage.

It's warm outside, you don't have to hide.

It's safe to show others who you are.
It's safe to live in your skin.
It's safe when people who don't know you judge you.
It's safe to let your heart exist out in the open.

It's sunny outside, no need to hide.

It's safe to feel deeply.
It's safe to be open.
It's safe to let others go.
It's safe to cry.
It's safe to feel hurt.

It's still beautiful outside, don't hide.

It's safe to get help.
It's safe to talk about small problems.
It's safe to let others know you.
It's safe to admit you're wrong.

You are safe in this life.
Lift your heart to the sky.

Be free.

—*Mary Carreon*

While many clients like to write their own invocation, others ask that I write one for them. I will often use the *Preparation* and *Integration* sessions as a chance to listen for the intention of the journey to focus in on the person's primary goal. I never know exactly what a person will see or hear in their *Exploration* session. However, I'm often surprised that the experience is exactly what they need. I also like to use the invocation to help the client settle in—as they leave the ordinary world behind and get comfortable in the unique healing spaces we have cultivated. When you meet with your therapist for your *Preparation* session, the two of you can discuss what type of invocation you'd like to use. Many therapists are more than happy to write an invocation based on what the two of you discuss. What follows is an actual invocation I've written for a client, which may be appropriate for you, too. Other clients prefer to have invocations from other writers be read to them. I've included other invocation examples from some wonderful experts in this space. These are just a few of the countless invocations out there. If you'd like to read or have one of these invocations read to you, mark the page. If you're writing your own invocation, these can also serve as inspiration.

THE EAGLE INVOCATION

As you settle into the zero-gravity chair and put the eyeshades on, just notice the place in the body you already feel the most relaxed. As you feel the body cocooned by the gravity blanket, you can know that you are physically safe . . . which can help you to trust, relax, and let go through this journey. And the locket of your mother's photo that's on your lap is a reminder of the inner mother within you. . . . Oh, sweet mother, who is always here . . . guiding and protecting you.

Your body already knows how to breathe, and many people take comfort in knowing that this medicine doesn't affect your body's basic functions—like the ones that keep you alive. And perhaps you can even thank the breath for giving you oxygen without you needing to think of it. Use the breath when you need it through this journey, but also know that there's no need to think about breathing. In this space, you are safe and supported.

You can thank parts of the mind for keeping you safe. . . . Even any apprehension, which, of course, is an emotional cousin of excitement . . . is a part of you that always keeps you alive. Imagine you're moving the part of you that's on high alert to the side of the room . . . and now, outside this room. Tell that part of you that it's okay to go offline now. You're okay. You're okay. It's okay to be open, to trust, and relax. Even hearing the sound of my voice, you can really just acknowledge how taken care of you are here . . . noticing the part of you that already feels at ease and peaceful . . . and imagining that this part of you is growing now. As the parts of you that have protected you soften and are disarmed, you make room for the Self—the seat of consciousness, the divine within. . . . And it's nice to know that the medicine will help you understand the Self in a deeper way. You are more than the parts of yourself that have kept you alive. Parts of your personality are not the same as you. You are the Self—the part of you that contains these parts.

And now, as you feel your sleeve being rolled up, and now, the medicine entering the body, . . . you can ask the medicine to show you what you need today. Remember your intention: How can I live in a way that is free? Boundless and courageous. One that is filled with self-love and compassion. Help me to live a life that is guided by Self and not ego. And may the parts of me realize that while they have protected me, they no longer need to do that. Medicine, show me something that will help me to understand the core of my barriers in a new way and for the parts to integrate so that they don't have to be at war anymore. Oh, sacred journey, help me to see what I need to do in my life to walk this path. Dear medicine, help me to know what it can feel like to fly like an eagle, free from earthly concerns . . .

> And so, you can fly now . . .
> with a sense of calm, cool, comfort.
> Trust, relax, and fly . . .
> Set yourself free . . .
> Soaring through this journey of your earthly life . . .
> And also connecting with something that this special world will bring you . . .
> Something greater than you've known before . . .
> Aligned with the Self . . .
> More meaningful . . .
> Or, maybe, more special or divine.
>
> And like an eagle who lives on this earth but can also soar to the heavens . . .
> May you live in this space, the blue sky that separates heaven and earth . . .
> The Self and the parts of you . . .
> These two worlds are more connected than you know.
> Find the healing elixir . . .
> that you can bring back to this world . . .
>
> This journey belongs to you now . . .
> It always has.

Trust, relax, and let go now . . .
Fly now . . .
Good journey . . .

—*Dr. Mike Dow*

* * *

CANYON RIVER CANOE ANALOGY

This analogy I share with you today provides a metaphor for thinking about the psychedelic experience you are about to journey on. It reflects the potential of this powerful medicine. The medicine allows us to explore amazing places that reflect the wonderful complexity of the human experience. Therapeutic work happens during the journey of self-exploration and healing.

This medicine has the potential to open many doors. It has the potential to also gently close doors that may cause excessive pain and suffering. Proper preparation and help with experienced guides are useful to help us to explore these doors. Working with psychedelic medicine can be compared to the skill of paddling a canoe down a river floating through a canyon. On this river, you may set out with companions who will help paddle with you to your destination. You are never alone on your journey with psychedelic medicines. Guides are here to help you relax. Please know that your environment is safe, and you will be supported in whatever ways are needed from people you trust. You can also invite with you, in your heart, the people who have helped you make your way to this point in time.

On the river, when you push off in your canoe from the shore, the banks gently rise beside you, guiding the direction of the journey. The banks are lush with trees, shrubs, and grass. It takes great courage to embark on this voyage, and the many people who have gone before you often feel nervous at the start. This is okay. It means this experience matters. You have committed to the journey, and the river will now take you on your way to your destination where you can safely carry your canoe away from the flowing water.

The analogy with psychedelic medicine is that once you take the medication, you are also committed to the journey and there is only one direction to go— which is down the river of time.

There are many factors that influence the experience of the canoe traveling down the river. One of them is the breeze, which can gently nudge you along or can come upstream, asking you to meet its energy.

Within the psychedelic journey the environment of the experience is analogous to the breeze. The music, eyeshades, and the setting of the room are all powerful and important parts of creating safety and a positive healing environment.

Another factor that influences the experience of canoeing in a canyon river is the fact that you have a paddle, as it is not just the breeze that influences where you go. You can paddle the canoe to the left or right of the river, and you can move around obstacles on your journey.

Within the psychedelic journey, the paddle is analogous to the fact that in some journeys you may be able to make choices about where in your mind you focus your attention. You may be able to pick and choose the parts of yourself you would like to explore. And in some journeys you may not have this choice. This is okay. There is no wrong or right path. Embrace what unfolds and welcome it with an open heart and mind.

On the river, there are times when the water flows faster and may become turbulent. You can be comforted by knowing that the guides are familiar with this river. There are life jackets to ensure everyone is safe and always above the water.

Within the psychedelic journey the life jacket is analogous to meditation and staying focused on breathing. A skillful person who uses psychedelic medicine will practice taking long, slow, deep breaths and focus on the sensations of breathing to relax and to induce a sense of calm, which allows the focus to remain on healing and presence.

Many Indigenous traditions believe that rivers have a spirit and offer wisdom to those willing to listen. Indigenous leaders with great experience encourage us to embrace what happens on this journey by saying "Thank you" and "Trust your own internal healer." Listening to the river is important when we paddle a canoe, and trusting the process is important when experiencing psychedelic medicine.

So, in preparation for your psychedelic healing journey, be reminded that you are safe, within a therapeutic room with support. Practice your slow, deep breathing to remain calm during this experience. You always have a guide with you to ensure safety. Trust your own inner healer, trust the medicine, and, no matter what may manifest, take a long, slow, deep breath and say "Thank you."

—Dr. Michael Verbora
Adapted from previous trainings

* * *

South

To the winds of the South
Great Serpent
Wrap your coils of light around us
Teach us to shed the past the way you shed your skin
To walk softly on the Earth
Teach us the Beauty Way

West

To the winds of the West
Mother Jaguar
Protect our medicine space
Teach us the way of peace, to live impeccably
Show us the way beyond death

North

To the winds of the North
Hummingbird, Grandmothers, and Grandfathers
Ancient Ones
Come and warm your hands by our fires
Whisper to us in the wind
We honor you who have come before us
And you who will come after us, our children's children

East

To the winds of the East
Great Eagle, Condor
Come to us from the place of the rising Sun
Keep us under your wing
Show us the mountains we only dare to dream of
Teach us to fly wing to wing with the Great Spirit

Mother Earth

We've gathered for the healing of all of your children
The Stone People, the Plant People
The four-legged, the two-legged, the creepy-crawlers
The finned, the furred, and the winged ones
All our relations

Father Sun

Father Sun, Grandmother Moon, to the Star Nations
Great Spirit, you who are known by a thousand names
And you who are the unnamable One
Thank you for bringing us together
And allowing us to sing the Song of Life

—Dr. Alberto Villoldo, The Four Winds

* * *

What if you could feel inner pulsating and see the colors of you?
What if you felt trapped in your body and couldn't move to the music you were
hearing and feeling . . . or could you?
But you weren't. Why? Judgment?
What if the whole world was waiting for you to dance or sing or be the most
fabulous you?
You're the one you've been waiting for, searching for . . .

So live.
And dance.
And feel it all.
Become one with nature . . . and this experience.
Float with the waves some moments.
And others, ride them—even when oceans fall from your eyes.
As you watch the flicker of a flame, become the fire and light up the sky so that
no darkness can survive.
Become one with the earth and melt into oneness.

Love her.
Love you.
Love all the parts of you.
You are her . . . and she is you, infinitely.
What will happen when there's no more longing?
When there's nothing missing?
You're whole.
You've arrived at you, the home that was always within.

—Dr. Jill Stocker

* * *

MY INVOCATION

Refer back to your Intention on page 99. How would you like to connect your intention to your invocation? Remember, you can either: (1) write your own invocation, (2) select an invocation from above or another source, or (3) ask your therapist to write an invocation for you. If you'd like to write your own invocation, you can write it here.

There are no right or wrong answers, but remember that you will be in a highly suggestible state. These will be the last words you hear before crossing the bridge from this ordinary world to the world of the ketamine journey. Open your heart, and ask for what you really need.

It can be helpful to keep your invocation positive. When possible, favor positive language over negative language. For example, say, "She is on a journey to reclaim her joy" instead of "She's been depressed for 10 years." As you may have noticed in the invocation above, I also tend to use softer language if there is a word with a slightly negative charge. Instead of *anxiety*, I used the word *apprehension*. Instead of "Get rid of the paralyzing fear," I used phrases and imagery like "Fly like an eagle, free of earthly concerns."

It can also be helpful to write poetically by using metaphors and rich imagery, because they are the language of the subconscious. Since ketamine is an amplifier of the subconscious, writing in this format is speaking the language of the medicine journey. You may want to write in the third person or try to limit the words *I* and *me*. *I*, *me*, and *myself* are words the ego uses to keep it separate from others and the world.

Your invocation can be anywhere from 15 seconds to a few minutes long when read. If you are receiving ketamine via an intramuscular injection at Field Trip, the medicine comes on within a few minutes. Thus, the invocation should be fairly short. If it's longer, ask your therapist to begin reading it before the medicine enters your body. If you are using sublingual ketamine at home, your invocation can be longer—since the medicine will take 10 to 15 minutes to begin working. You can either read the invocation to yourself or e-mail it to your therapist so he or she can read it to you remotely.

Invocation for my first *Exploration* session:

4. Consider Special Objects

Many people find it helpful to bring special objects that help them connect to their intention. There are no right or wrong answers in terms of what to bring, and nor are you required to bring something.

Is there an object that helps you feel safe and supported? If so, you can place the object on your lap and reach for it when you feel lost. This can be especially helpful if using the Field Trip at Home™ protocol. The physical comfort of this object can replace your therapist's hand-holding—which is typically offered to clients at Field Trip.

Is there an object that conceptualizes your main goal? If you are grieving, you may want to bring a photo of your loved one to place by your chair. Other clients like to wear an article of clothing that belonged to their loved one. If your highest, healthiest self is going to return to the diet that heals your body as it gives up bingeing or processed foods, perhaps you can bring your favorite healthy food to put on the table next to you (and eat it when the medicine wears off). If you are in recovery, you can bring a chip to be reminded of the wisdom of your program. If you want to reconnect with your calling, bring or wear something that represents service—like your first pair of scrubs if you're a nurse and felt called to this line of work. If you want to return to the childlike wonder you've lost, perhaps a toy from your childhood.

Is there an object that has religious or spiritual significance to you? Our role as therapists is not to be your pastor, rabbi, guru, or spiritual leader. However, we also recognize that true healing must address all of the bio-psycho-social-spiritual parts within us. Thus, we are here to hold space for your most deeply held beliefs.

Some clients have brought in angel card decks and they pull a card just before their journey. Others have brought prayer cards, crystals, or prayer beads. If you are not spiritual in any way, that's fine. Any object that means something to you is appropriate to bring in. This healing journey is yours. We are here to hold space for your healing—so that the medicine can bring forth the inner healing intelligence that has always been there.

5. What to Expect

Now it's time to talk about the simple logistics you should be aware of. These tips are more important than people realize. Make this journey special and sacred. In the list below, you'll find simple tips like arriving on time. These may sound like common-sense tips that apply to any appointment, but we'd like to remind you that this journey is no ordinary appointment. Things that wouldn't necessarily affect you can sometimes have a profound effect on your journey.

Ketamine is an amplifier of the subconscious that also affects levels of multiple neurotransmitters. If you rush out the door and then get caught in traffic, you're flooding the body with stress hormones like adrenaline. Ketamine lifts levels of the "upper" dopamine in your brain. The adrenaline mixed with dopamine could potentially color your journey and bring anxiety-provoking imagery to the surface.

One client recently was reminded of this when he had a huge fight with his mom just before his session. Since his previous five *Exploration* sessions were all deep, beautiful, and positive, he was surprised that this journey was colored by tension, anger, and darkness. It was only *after* his journey ended that he told me about the fight. If he would have told me before the session, I would have encouraged him to reschedule. While *Exploration* sessions are an opportunity to heal deep interpersonal wounds, we also don't want you to take the medicine while still actively in the fight-or-flight response just after a fight ends.

Try to avoid work calls. Don't take work calls the morning of your *Exploration* session. Better yet: Don't take any calls at all. If something unavoidable comes up like a huge fight with your spouse, be honest with your therapist and, if necessary, reschedule. Small snafus like a bit of traffic are unavoidable and are unlikely to color your journey. However, the biggest fight you've had in a year may affect the journey in a negative way. While challenging experiences often provide an opportunity for deep healing, we also don't want to prime the subconscious with deep negativity.

Some of the rules below aren't absolutes, but some are. You should absolutely fast for a minimum of four hours to prevent nausea/vomiting and to enhance the effects of the ketamine. Also, you are not permitted to drive after sessions under any circumstances.

However, if you are prescribed a benzodiazepine to take daily and you need it, it's usually not an issue taking it if you're honest with us during your screening. One client was pleasantly surprised by how much deeper her journey was when she avoided Xanax, prescribed to take as needed, in the days before her *Exploration* sessions. In the days leading up to her *Exploration* sessions, she practiced yoga, did breathing exercises, and took walks in nature. She didn't need the Xanax and reported that her *Exploration* session felt "twice as deep" compared to previous ones. She and her therapist noticed a profound reduction in anxiety halfway through her initial course of six *Exploration* sessions, so she worked with her pre-scriber to wean off the Xanax. Not all clients will titrate off their medication. For those who take them, ketamine tends to make them work better. Use this journey as a time to become very intentional with what you want.

Some medications require communication among providers. Since ketamine tends to spike your blood pressure, we'll usually have clients skip their stimulant like Adderall on the day of the *Exploration* session. Antidepressants that are taken daily like SSRIs and SNRIs are generally fine to take the day of an *Exploration* session. Ketamine is generally a very safe medicine with very few drug-drug interactions. Always check with your prescriber and be honest with our staff so we can keep you safe and ensure your journey helps you heal.

Preparation Checklist

- Please arrive on time and avoid stress or rushing on the day of your appointment, so be aware of traffic conditions.

- Aim for a minimum of 8 to10 hours of sleep the night before a ketamine session.

- Fast for at least four hours prior to a ketamine session.

- Avoid alcohol, cannabis, opioids, NSAIDs (such as aspirin or ibuprofen), stimulants, sedative hypnotics, and muscle relaxants for 48 hours prior to a ketamine session.

- Bring your rescue inhaler, blood pressure medication, or any other emergency medication, if applicable.

- Refrain from using any other psychedelics for seven days prior to and after a ketamine session.

- Arrange for a ride home.

- Wear loose, comfortable clothing for a ketamine session.

- Bring your patient care bag with journal, pen, eyeshades, and slippers if they are not provided for you.

- Take time to connect with your intentions for seeking this treatment.

- Complete the questionnaire that will be sent by our clinic.

- Identify a support person you can reach out to if needed after leaving the clinic.

- Identify relaxing/calming behaviors in which to engage if you feel activated post-session.

- Take emotional and physical care of yourself before and after each ketamine session—your time in treatment is a special time and taking care of yourself helps maximize your experience. Activities might include these:

  - Light exercise

  - Eating healthy, nourishing meals (nothing out of the ordinary)

  - Light housekeeping so you can come back to a clean home—no dirty dishes, clean bed/sheets, comfortable clothes, and rest areas

  - Listening to relaxing music

  - Using breathing to relax or process emotions, or practice mindfulness, yoga, or other relaxation techniques

  - Journaling

  - Taking walks or spending time in nature

  - Talking with supportive friends and family (it's not the time to have upsetting or stressful conversations)

  - Avoiding negative media (TV, movies, social media, podcasts, etc.)

  - Reconnecting with your intention for the session, as discussed with your therapist

6. Prepare Mind, Body, and Spirit for the Journey

It can be helpful to be very specific and intentional when preparing the mind, body, and spirit for the Ketamine-Assisted Psychotherapy journey. The general guidelines listed above are a terrific place to start. Now, ask yourself if there is anything special *you* would like to do to prepare *your* mind, body, and spirit.

What centers and calms *your* mind? Do you have a favorite walk or bike path? Who are the people who help you feel supported? On the other hand, are there any people or conversations you should avoid during the days leading up to your *Exploration* session? While this journey often helps people to eventually resolve long-standing issues, it's best not to open up any wounds during this preparatory phase. Can you put away messages on your work e-mail? Can you find a babysitter or pet sitter so you can have some time for meditation and journaling? Take a moment to consider how you will prepare *your* mind.

I will prepare my mind by

_____

_____

_____

How do you feel best in your body? What's your diet like? Some Ketamine-Assisted Psychotherapy practitioners recommend a whole-food, plant-based diet in the days leading up to the *Exploration* session. If you are following a Mediterranean, anti-inflammatory, or autoimmune protocol diet that's essential to your healing, then that's a healthy choice as well. No matter what you are eating, can you choose foods consciously and eat mindfully? Are you practicing good sleep hygiene and turning off all screens at night to prepare the body for deep rest? Do you stop eating three hours before bedtime? How about exercise and movement? What helps you feel grounded in your body?

I will prepare my body by

_____

_____

_____

What speaks to your spirit? Do you pray or have any religious practices? How about an existing transcendental or mindfulness meditation practice? These ongoing practices tend to make ketamine journeys deeper, and ketamine journeys then enhance these practices. Does spending time in nature ground and soothe your soul? Are there any rituals you use? Can you clear your home or the previous chapters of your life with sage or incense? Are there any religious or spiritual books that help you connect with your spirit? How do you get in touch with God, spirit, soul, higher power, or wise self?

I will prepare my spirit by

_____

_____

_____

7. Read "The Guest House" by Rumi

This poem by Rumi is a reminder to greet anything and everything you encounter in this journey with an open door, open heart, and open mind. Have a curious, welcoming, and nonjudgmental attitude at every step of this journey. As much as we prepare you for the road ahead, it is highly likely that something unexpected will surface. Ketamine journeys are like snowflakes: No two are the same. It's not uncommon for your *Exploration* sessions to each have a very different feeling, tone, or message. Greet every message or lesson at the door with a smile. After all, everything—including the words you're now reading and any images you see in your *Exploration* that may come up—have, as Rumi said, been sent as a "guide from beyond."

The Guest House
This being human is a guest house.
Every morning a new arrival.

A joy, a depression, a meanness,
some momentary awareness comes
as an unexpected visitor.

Welcome and entertain them all!
Even if they're a crowd of sorrows,
who violently sweep your house
empty of its furniture,
still, treat each guest honorably.

He may be clearing you out
for some new delight.

The dark thought, the shame, the malice,
meet them at the door laughing,
and invite them in.

Be grateful for whoever comes,
because each has been sent
as a guide from beyond.

* * *

Bring all of your responses from the activities in this chapter to your *Preparation* session with your therapist. Your therapist will help you deepen the work you've done here. Like any talk therapy session, it will also be a time to dialogue and process your experience. This session will also be a time to ask any specific questions about the road ahead. The therapeutic relationship you will form, or already have, with your therapist will guide your journey, so lean on it. Know that you are cared for and supported. In terms of the way you feel, know that there are no right or wrong ways to feel about this journey. Greet any feelings with an open curiosity, and trust that the medicine and this work will synergistically bring forth the healing *you* need.

CHAPTER 11

THE KAP WORKBOOK: THE EXPLORATION SESSION

This chapter is your guide to your *Exploration* sessions, the ones that include the administration of ketamine. Everything you have read in this book, the activities you completed in the last chapter, and your *Preparation* session with your therapist has prepared you for the journey ahead. While the specific goals of the *Exploration* sessions vary from person to person, they tend to go directly to the root causes of a person's suffering by providing insight, understanding, and monumental shifts in perspective. We often tell people that one *Exploration* session can uncover what would take months or years in talk therapy. Whereas traditional talk therapy often peels back an onion one layer at a time, an *Exploration* session can peel back multiple layers in just a few hours. One common goal of these complementary practices: to allow hidden parts to emerge. Should you return to weekly talk therapy after your *Exploration* sessions, you will likely find that your KAP experience will enhance and deepen your ongoing work.

For clients with PTSD, the *Exploration* sessions may involve reprocessing trauma while boosting serotonin levels—leading to a general feeling of safety. For clients with treatment-resistant depression, the *Exploration* sessions may help turn down the default mode network (DMN) associated with rumination and boost dopamine—leading to a feeling of optimism. Or, it may provide a mystical experience that changes the way they see themselves in this world—adding greater meaning to their everyday life. For clients with anxiety, the *Exploration* sessions may help them see or understand the root of their fear—leading to a feeling of peace.

Or there may be some archetype (see Chapter 12) that tells them they will always be safe and supported. For clients grieving a loss, the *Exploration* sessions may involve seeing their loved one in a different form—leading to a feeling that he or she is okay. Ketamine can simultaneously achieve these goals biochemically as it changes the brain—psychologically and spiritually—through images, visions, and archetypes, which are the language of the subconscious. As you can probably gather from these examples, the way the healing manifests varies widely from person to person.

Now that you've done your prep work, your role in your *Exploration* sessions is exactly what it sounds like: to explore. You'll be exploring your personal unconscious, the collective unconscious, your past, the universe, your spirit, and the part of you that is separate from ego.

The way the human brain categorizes known objects or experiences prevents the need for time-consuming analysis of them—which allows you to quickly turn your attention to dangerous ones that require attention. While this efficient processing keeps you alive, it can also make life feel mundane. Your brain's top-down processing mechanism is like a sorting machine, sending down information based on what it's learned to categorize the incoming sensory information from the bottom up. You could say that the intersection of these signals is when you experience consciousness—the moment you know the fragrant and soft red object is a rose.

But if you turn off that sorting machine, would you be able to see things in a new way? Just because these organized, ordinary ways of perceiving are the brain's default way of making sense of the world, does it mean that this is the only "real" way to be? Similarly, what if you could take in all the information about yourself without repressing, splitting, displacing, subjugating, compartmentalizing, minimizing, projecting, denying, or somatizing unmet psychological needs into the physical body? Would this help you cultivate true integration of all parts of yourself and strive for true self-love?

What would it be like if you could experience every rose as if you're seeing it for the first time? Would you stop and appreciate it with the childlike sense of wonder you lost along the way? Would openness, awe, and wonder replace a gray, been-there-done-that attitude? Is the rose you see a symbol for something in your life? Is the rose your passionate heart that needs to open up again? Ketamine journeys tend to be rich with meaning. The time has come to simply stay open to everything your inner healing intelligence has to show you via the administration of the incredible medicine known as ketamine.

This chapter includes the following activities:

1. Determining Your Dose

2. Optimizing the Set and Setting

3. Understanding the Role of Music

4. Listening to the Flight Instructions and Your Intention

5. Taking the Medicine

1. Determining Your Dose

Your health-care professionals determine a ketamine dose that is both safe and effective for you. However, your dose should be a collaborative decision between you and your provider. It's helpful to understand the way different doses feel subjectively. Unlike IV ketamine clinics that use fairly standard dosing based on a person's weight, Ketamine-Assisted Psychotherapy uses a more personalized dose. We have found that a person's personality traits, life history, previous psychotherapy history, and experience with psychedelics should all be considered when determining the optimal dose.

For example, people who score high on "openness" using the popular Big Five personality test, tend to be able to tolerate larger doses right away. That being said, we also know that these journeys can increase openness in people who feel anxious or afraid—functioning as a type of exposure therapy. Thus, perhaps it's the person who's *not* very open who will benefit most from high-dose sessions. If that sounds scary, no need to worry. With Ketamine-Assisted Psychotherapy, we can slowly and incrementally increase your dose with every session—in the same way that cognitive behavioral therapy moves slowly via graded exposure.

On top of these psychological concerns, we also must consider the physical body. If your blood pressure is on the high side of our accepted range, we will likely want to start with a low-dose *Exploration* session to see how ketamine affects your blood pressure before moving to high-dose work. As you can see, dosing is a decision that requires weighing many factors. Personalized dosing allows us to tailor the medicine to your goals and history while simultaneously pairing it with the type of psychotherapy needed.

Your personalized goals also affect how many *Exploration* sessions you will need and how closely they need to be stacked. People with untreated, severe trauma who frequently dissociate may benefit from low-dose sessions that allow for psychotherapy throughout the *Exploration* sessions. In this case, stacking the sessions closely together may be less important (e.g., three *Exploration* sessions over three months with *Integration* sessions in between). Another person with severe depression, no history of trauma, and many positive experiences with psychedelics may have better effects with high-dose sessions. In this case, stacking the *Exploration* sessions is more important (e.g., six *Exploration* sessions within a three-week time frame). When it comes to mood disorders, we ideally want to do the next *Exploration* session before the lifted mood falls back to its baseline. After the first *Exploration* session, the mood will sometimes lift for 24 hours. By the third *Exploration* session, the mood improvement will often last days or weeks. Thus, it's probably more important to stack sessions one and two within one week than it is to stack sessions five and six closely together. Someone who is feeling stuck after a divorce and experiencing mixed anxiety and depression may need only two low- to medium-dose *Exploration* sessions scheduled a few weeks apart.

While studies provide guidelines in terms of what works for most people, we like to think of each client as a "N-of-1" trial. In layman's terms, that means that *your* response is the most important guideline. While research has shown that six *Exploration* sessions is effective for treatment-resistant depression, six may not be your magic number. You may need only four *Exploration* sessions. If you start with low-dose work for two sessions, you may need a total of seven *Exploration* sessions. Another variable that needs to be considered—how sensitive you are to the medicine. The only way to know for sure is to assess your subjective experience at different doses, which for most clients will slowly taper up with every *Exploration* session. Also, Ketamine-Assisted Psychotherapy includes *Integration* sessions in between your *Exploration* sessions, so you'll be getting the benefits of both the medicine and psychotherapy. Because we're combining two proven treatments, there tends to be more variability compared to IV ketamine clinics that offer medicine with no concurrent psychotherapy.

The dosage guidelines below give typical ranges. Remember: One dose may feel like a medium-dose session to one person and a low-dose session to another. Tracking your mood throughout the protocol is the best way to determine your ideal dose and rhythm, and your therapist may use tools like the PHQ-9 to track depressive symptoms, the GAD-7 to track symptoms of anxiety disorders, or the Mystical Experiences Questionnaire to assess your subjective experience of the journey itself. There tends to be a correlation between how mystical a ketamine journey feels and objective measures of depression and anxiety. The takeaway here is this:

Throughout the initial series of *Exploration* sessions, we home in on the optimal dose and interval for you, how many initial *Exploration* sessions you'll need, and how well the *Explorations* sessions are at healing the root cause of what's ailing you.

If you choose a low-dose *Exploration* session, you probably won't fully "leave the room" and your ego will stay fairly intact. Low-dose sessions are sometimes called psycholytic, mind-loosening, empathogenic, subpsychedelic, or hypnodelic sessions. In this type of session, you'll likely just feel a bit warm and floaty with very mild dissociation. Challenging moments or the novel experience of ego dissolution are rare in low-dose *Exploration* sessions. The downside to low-dose work is that ketamine's benefits are somewhat dose-dependent, so people with very severe mental illness will likely need higher doses for maximum benefit. In low-dose *Exploration* sessions, your heart will likely feel open and your defenses will be lowered. This type of session allows for psychotherapy, hypnosis, trauma reprocessing, or guided imagery throughout the entire *Exploration* session if needed—since you'll be present enough to understand and communicate. One or two low-dose *Exploration* sessions are also a good place to start for people who feel very nervous about ketamine before working their way up to medium- or high-dose sessions.

People seeking transcendent, transpersonal (beyond the personal psyche) experiences or who are suffering with more severe mental illness should consider medium- to high-dose sessions. In this type of session, you will cross the bridge from the ordinary world to the special, psychedelic world of a ketamine journey—encountering a more complete loss of ego and its defenses with rich visuals, leaving the body, seeing loved ones you've lost, having mystical experiences, accessing lost memories, journeying to other lands or space, feeling totally at one with all living beings, a feeling of being a single point of consciousness, and losing any sense of ordinary time or space. You will "leave the room" and will often, at some point, have no awareness of where you are. You will be at one with the experience.

Concurrent psychotherapy isn't possible during the deepest part of the journey, because people aren't able to understand what's being said. In fact, they should allow the music to be the therapist. It's helpful to remember that there are three therapists in the room with you at all times: your therapist, the music, and you (via your inner therapist or "inner healing intelligence"). While many people are silent in medium- and high-dose *Exploration* sessions, some do talk. In these cases, the therapist is there to write down what is said. That's important, since people often won't remember what they say at higher doses—and the statements can be quite profound. Ideally, we want to find the dose that is high enough to give you a mystical experience but low enough that you can remember most or all of your journey. If you don't remember your journey, the ketamine will still improve your neurochemistry and act as an antidepressant. But you'll lose some of the psycho-social-spiritual benefits and profound aha moments that can change the way you see yourself or the universe. Remember: The doses we use are lower than when ketamine is used as anesthesia. Rather than putting you to sleep, our goal is waking you up to your life.

Most in-clinic sessions will deliver the medicine via a quick and fairly painless intramuscular injection that, unlike ketamine IV, doesn't require a needle to stay inserted through the journey (which, of course, tends to make the journey more peaceful). Intramuscular ketamine has a 93 percent bioavailability with a rapid onset.[1] Intramuscular ketamine carries a lower risk of nausea/vomiting compared to ketamine taken by mouth.

If you are going through an at-home protocol, you will take ketamine orally. The bioavailability ranges from 17 percent to 29 percent, which we adjust for when calculating your dose.[2] Since the ketamine is absorbed mostly in the mouth (sublingually and transmucosally), you'll have to hold the medicine in your mouth for up to 15 minutes before swallowing. The onset is much slower compared to intramuscular injection—which also makes the *Exploration* session longer. Whether you're using intramuscular injection or oral ketamine, the anti-nausea drug Zofran can be administered before or after the ketamine to prevent or treat nausea/vomiting. Tell your provider if you have a history of nausea so they can provide you with Zofran. We also offer people ginger or mint tea just after their journey, which is also helpful. Unlike IV ketamine that delivers a steady state of ketamine over the course of the session (typically 0.5 milligrams per kilogram), intramuscular injection delivers all the medicine to you at the beginning of the *Exploration* session, which can make it feel more like a true and mystical "trip." It's usually given in one single dose, but in the first *Exploration* session, we will sometimes use split dosing—delivering a booster dose within 10 minutes after the first injection. If you're using oral ketamine, the booster dose is usually given within 15 to 20 minutes after first placing the medicine in your mouth. Booster dosing can help people get comfortable with the way the medicine feels before they decide whether or not they want to go deeper.

Consider a person who is very nervous about taking ketamine for the first time. In the first *Exploration* session, we may start with a lower dose of around 25 milligrams via intramuscular injection. We'll check in 5 to 10 minutes later and ask if the client wants to go deeper. If the client says they want to go just a little bit deeper, we'll add a booster dose of 10 milligrams. If they tolerated that well, we may then offer that client an injection of 40 milligrams—a slightly larger total amount of medicine—in one dose for the second *Exploration* session. Most clients gradually increase their dose with every *Exploration* session until we find the optimal dose that also accounts for tolerance.

The way you feel about dosing is a vital piece in determining your dose.

Ketamine Dosage Guidelines: Exploration Sessions

- **LOW:** 15–35 milligrams intramuscular injection, or 45–100 milligrams for oral route
  Description: Warm, mildly dissociative or "floaty," but usually won't "leave the room." Light visuals or seeing a gradual "fade to black" or sense of floating in space. Feelings of compassion; ego/defenses are weakened but present. Awareness of where and who you are usually remains intact, concurrent psychotherapy (e.g., hypnosis, imagery, trauma reprocessing) usually possible throughout the session.

- **MEDIUM:** 35–75 milligrams intramuscular injection, or 100–200 milligrams for oral route
  Description: Begins to act as a psychedelic, visuals become intense and colorful, travel into other times and memories, begin to leave the body or "leave the room." Ego is mostly offline, flashbacks to memories, trauma may resurface. Concurrent psychotherapy is usually possible only when the client is "coming back" into the room.

- **HIGH:** 75+ milligrams intramuscular injection, or 200+ milligrams for oral route
  Description: Transpersonal (beyond the personal psyche) and transcendental experiences, out-of-body experiences, loss of identity, visits from mystical beings or loved ones. Total oneness with the universe, ego death, reexperiencing the birth process, or experiencing being reborn, can mimic near-death experiences as the dose increases. Concurrent psychotherapy is usually possible only as the client is coming back into the room.

Now that I understand ketamine dosing, I am feeling _____

and think I would benefit most from a _____ *-dose session.*

2. Optimizing Set and Setting

Set refers to your mindset or what's happening within you during a ketamine journey—including your thoughts, feelings, mood, expectations, and how ready you're feeling now that you've had your *Preparation* session. *Setting* refers to your physical surroundings and what's happening outside of you—including the feel of the room, the way the zero-gravity chair feels, the social support between you and your therapist, and the culturally accepted norms of what is real. Both set and setting have a profound effect on your journey, so it's important to be cognizant of them. Ketamine-Assisted Psychotherapy is done with closed eyes, with music, and with light-blocking eyeshades, which helps enhance the medicine's effects and allows you to go in.

The importance of *set and setting* was noted in the psychedelic research that took place in America during the 1950s and '60s from research being done primarily on LSD and psilocybin-assisted psychotherapy. In 1958, a World Health Organization report on psychedelics noted that psychedelics' benefits were determined by carefully controlled environmental factors.[3] In 1964, Timothy Leary made the phrase *set and setting* famous when he published his book *The Psychedelic Experience*. Leary was influenced by the psychedelic research going on at the time, his own work, and writings given to him by writer Aldous Huxley from Paris's Hashish Club. This club was made up of a famous group of scientists and literary elite who dedicated themselves to hashish, a potent form of marijuana that can cause hallucinations, in the mid-1800s. "Tranquil frame of mind and body" was recommended to ensure a trip was pleasurable and to prevent bad trips.[4]

Everything we do in Ketamine-Assisted Psychotherapy is designed to promote "tranquil frame of mind and body," and this includes optimizing set (or mindset) and setting. Clients coming into a Field Trip center will immediately notice that the setting probably feels more like they're walking into a yoga retreat center than a doctor's office. The color palette of the design, the fractals from nature displayed on the walls, the soothing music we play in the reception area, the zero-gravity loungers in the treatment rooms, and the noise-canceling headphones are all designed to enhance set and setting.

During the session, your therapist will be sitting next to you. Be sure to discuss supportive touch during your journey before the medicine is given to you. If you'd like, your therapist can hold your hand when needed at any point during the journey. Give verbal consent for this before the journey begins. During the journey, simply reach for your therapist's hand at any time and hold it for as long as you'd like. Some will find this has a calming effect on their mindset. When your journey is over, we will bring you nourishing food, water, and tea. Since they've fasted for four or more hours, many people are quite hungry after the journey. Peppermint tea, ginger tea, fruit, and easy-to-digest snacks can help ease the stomach.

If you are using an at-home protocol, you can optimize set and setting in the same way. This work is best done in a space where you feel safe, supported, and stress-free, so stay away from rooms that your mind associates with work. Use colors, fabrics, and cushions that will optimize your journey. Although you may not be aware of it, your subconscious picks up on subtle cues. For example, research has shown that most people feel better in rooms with soft edges and round curves,[5] so bring softness into your room with blankets and pillows. If there are plants, greenery, or even photos of nature handy, put them around you. Your physical surroundings contribute to the literal container for your healing—just as your relationship with your therapist provides an energetic one. Since physical touch isn't possible with at-home sessions, consider bringing an object that helps you feel safe. You can place the object by your side or in your lap.

You'll want to be either in a very comfortable reclining chair or lying down. Couches, beds, yoga mats, or floor cushions can all make for some very comfortable places for this work. While rare, vomiting is possible—so have a trash can nearby, too. Have nourishing food, water, and tea within reach to eat after the journey comes to an end. The lighting should be soft and very dim so that when you take the eyeshades off, you'll have a smooth transition. If you identified any special objects you'd like to have in the last chapter, have them with you. You can either hold them or create an altar, placing the objects on a table nearby. Have your eyeshades and music ready to go. You can use any comfortable light-blocking sleep mask or the Mindfold brand eye mask. Know that set and setting are another important piece of your special journey.

3. Understand the Role of Music

Throughout the history of psychedelics, music has played an integral role using drum beats, bowls, and all sorts of sounds designed to enhance—not distract from—the experience. Music's role cannot be overstated. Besides the drug's effects, we can argue music is the most influential part of the psychedelic—and ketamine—journey. So this means plugging into your favorite playlist isn't necessarily therapeutic when under the ketamine influence. Instead, music selection becomes key for a desired outcome.

Instead of conventional music that you might listen to, we suggest music or playlists designed to facilitate psychedelic experiences. Wavepaths is generally recognized as the leading provider of music for psychedelic therapies, but there are a range of options available from specific artists such as East Forest and Jon Hopkins, playlists specifically compiled on Spotify by therapists, or you can find a wide range of supportive music through our Field Trip app.

Sounds of Discovery: How Music Becomes a Ketamine Companion
Interview with Mendel Kaelen, Founder of Wavepaths

What have you learned about why music is a key part of a psychedelic journey?

Music has the capacity to facilitate an experience because the music is perceived in much more detail and closeness, and because of the heightened hyper-associativity going on in the brain. So it's a blending of the senses. Every sound in a psychedelic experience, whether that's with ketamine or MDMA, is becoming a world in itself. Music provides structure in the absence of structure.

When it comes to ketamine, there seems to be a trait of being "in the moment," a great sense of zooming in, and the sound becomes more granular and more detailed. It almost seems that the continuity in music or the usual compositional structures don't matter as much with ketamine as compared to other psychedelics. Therefore, we want to think about the microstructures in the music. This is why tone color, for example, is such an important part of our research. In an altered state of consciousness, the subtle harmonics and the rhythms become dominant forms that your sense of hearing tunes in to.

What led you to get into this field of study, and what are some of the pivotal studies that show music becomes an active participant in the process?

This is a topic I am incredibly passionate about. I've dedicated my life to understanding this. What I've learned is that music in psychedelic therapy with ketamine, or any scientific medicine, is not just background music. It plays an active therapeutic role. You can really guide the experience into all sorts of different directions and therapeutic processes, and help to deepen that, and help to facilitate change, in essence. That's why I called one of my papers "The Hidden Therapist," because we're finding music as a therapeutic companion. It's the third therapist in the room.

I became a researcher working with psychedelics at Imperial College of London, first a master's student, then a Ph.D., then a postdoc. Very early on at the beginning of my Ph.D., I realized everyone was using music in psychedelic therapy trials, but there was zero research on why we use music in the first place, and how the psychedelics and the music interact to facilitate these experiences. I wanted to learn how you can best work with music from patient to patient to support their therapeutic process.

126

Of course, there's much more historical lineage there when it comes to music and psychedelics that I believe should also be acknowledged. Music is a central component in any psychedelic ceremony you can think of worldwide, whether it's ibogaine ceremonies in Africa or peyote ceremonies of Native Americans or ayahuasca ceremonies. Anthropologists like Marlene Dobkin de Rios soon realized music played a major role in every single psychedelic ceremony that she was studying.

When I was a researcher at Imperial, I saw firsthand how therapists were struggling with music selection, and I noticed a real knowledge gap in understanding why certain pieces work the way they do for certain patients. Recognizing that knowledge gap and also the complexity in understanding both music and psychedelics, eventually led to Wavepaths.

When you look at how other cultures have used music with psychedelics, the shaman, as a facilitator and master of the ceremony, always has a toolkit available to influence the experience. A very important component of the toolkit has always been musical instruments. There are other tools as well, like incense, but musical instruments are always present. Typically, there are only a small number of musical instruments that one may say are archetypal for the shaman, like shamanic drumming, or rattles.

Rather than copying that into the present and saying, "Okay, the modern care provider also needs a shamanic drum or a rattle," the deeper and more important question is What music is best suited for all the states of consciousness? That is really our mission at Wavepaths.

How do you decide what kind of music works best for various conditions, like depression for example?

Psychedelics are an experiential form of therapy. I think it has to do with the fact that psychedelics primarily work through facilitating experiences that have significant personal meaning. So we're talking about facilitating new meanings and significant personal meaning, whereas the classical psychiatric model is devoid of that. It's based on a more purely mechanistic understanding of the brain, which is not necessarily totally wrong, but it's also not complete enough. There's something missing there in our understanding of mental health and how we can facilitate change.

Ketamine can facilitate a range of different experiences. There are lots of different experiences you can have when you're in an altered state of consciousness. But there are certain qualities in the experience that are most consistently associated with therapeutic improvements. Those qualities have to do with peak experiences, having mystical experiences, having personal insights, or having autobiographical cathartic experiences, and there are emotional release experiences. If you look at what all these experiences have in common, they are significantly personally meaningful.

Research suggests that psychedelic therapy can be defined or conceptualized as a model in which we aim to provide a climate for the patient that is favorable to experience new things about oneself. Now what does music have to do with all of this? How can music deepen these processes? How can music be used to increase the likelihood for a desired experience? First, what we have found is that music is able to facilitate these kinds of experiences with a higher likelihood than if music wasn't there.

How would you tailor this to someone, let's say, who has depression?

We are studying a phenomena called "the musical personality," which identifies acoustic compositional qualities of every listener. In other words, if we enhance the instrumentations, the acoustic properties, the compositional qualities, the genre preferences of an individual, and we use that in our filtering algorithm and our music selection procedures, there is a higher likelihood for that music to be personally resonating with the listener, and thereby increase the likelihood for these peak experiences to occur, for example. So that's one component to it.

The other component is related to the patient's condition. For depression, you may have two scenarios: First, it may be therapeutic to deepen the feelings of depression. The therapeutic wisdom behind this would be to learn the best way to get out of depression is to go through it. Music, then, can convey sadness and hopelessness back to the listener to bring the experience of depression more to the forefront to be dealt with.

Another path for using music and psychedelics to treat depression is to help relieve depression symptoms, to feel bliss and joy and to feel all of those experiences that have been unavailable for so long. So the sounds may feel lighter, uplifting, and positive.

Music provides direction, guiding the experience into a certain direction. So using music in psychedelic therapy makes psychedelic therapy a directive therapy. Can we provide direction in a person-centered way? Can we provide direction in a way that respects the autonomy, the integrity, and the condition of the patient, as well as the language that the patient speaks musically? Yes, and that's what we're doing at Wavepaths.

4. Listening to the Flight Instructions and Your Intention

The following may be read to you by your therapist at the beginning of your *Exploration* session. Listen to these suggestions with a receptive and open mind, heart, and spirit.

1. Every journey has a beginning, a middle, and an end.
2. You will come back.
3. Trust the process, trust the medicine, trust your inner organic healing intelligence, trust the therapy relationship.

4. Approach the journey with a "beginner's mindset" and curiosity.

5. Approach the journey like an anthropologist and an archaeologist.

6. Relax your critical mind so that you are not analyzing what you are experiencing or wondering why something is or is not coming up in the session.

7. Trust that whatever comes up in a session needs to come up, even if you do not fully understand it.

8. Trust that your inner healing intelligence would not bring up more than you can effectively handle or integrate.

9. When something beautiful or magical emerges, move toward it, connect with it, allow yourself to melt into it; when something is challenging, scary, confusing, or disturbing, in a similar way, move toward it with curiosity and inquiry.

10. When approaching challenging experiences (or appearances, forms, beings, or phenomena) ask what they are there to teach you and/or to show you, and if you can thank them for whatever is shared.

11. Keep moving (letting the music guide you and merge with you) and exploring and entering different spaces or terrains so that if you see doors, open them. If you see staircases, go up them. If you see planets, explore them. If you see bodies of water, go into them. If you see windows, jump through.

12. Imagine the music is holding your hand. Lean into the music.

13. Seeing is not believing in your journey space, but seeing is becoming and believing is through becoming.

14. Learn to use the breath to explore, inquire, and go deeper into experiences.

15. Ask for help whenever you need it in whatever form feels appropriate. Physical support, grounding, anchoring, and encouragement are available.

After reading these general flight instructions to you, your therapist will then read your specific intention you selected or wrote in the last chapter.

5. Taking the Medicine

There is nothing left to say except: Have a good journey.

CHAPTER 12

THE KAP WORKBOOK: THE INTEGRATION SESSION

While *Integration* sessions are stand-alone sessions that usually take place a day or two after your first, second, fourth, and sixth *Exploration* sessions, the process of integration is fluid. It begins as soon as the ketamine journey comes to an end and continues for the rest of your life.

It can be helpful to make this transition a smooth one, so don't abruptly take off the headphones and eyeshades. Take time to fully come back into the body, this world, and this room. Reflect on what message the journey is giving you today. Most people will immediately begin processing the experience with their therapist, though others like to stay silent. Usually you'll have some time to begin processing your experience in the treatment room with your therapist.

Of course you'll have more time to fully make sense of your experience in the *Integration* session in a day or two. At Field Trip, we also have integration lounges that clients can move to where they can continue to reflect, journal, or draw after they leave the individual treatment rooms. If you'd like, you can use this book as your journal. If you'd prefer, we also provide clients with a blank journal and colored pencils to write or draw.

Integration is different for every person. Here are the activities in this chapter:

1. Post-Journey Journal

2. At-Home Integration Activities

3. Additional Integration Exercises

If you think of *Exploration* sessions like a dream, it's also important to make sense of what you experienced. Like dreams, much of the material can soon be forgotten if it's not immediately verbalized to your therapist or written down. This is especially true in medium- and high-dose sessions.

The journal below is a template you can use to write down your experience. First, there is a space to answer three main considerations: the most important message you received, how you can heed this message in the ordinary world of your waking life, and what you'd like to make sense of in your *Integration* session with your therapist.

Then, you'll see two columns. On the left, there's a column titled "What I experienced." On the right is a column titled "What it means." We recommend writing down as many things as possible on the left-hand side under "What I experienced." Again, it can be easy to forget parts of the journey when this isn't done. It can be helpful to use an unfiltered stream-of-consciousness writing style when filling out this side. Many of the experiences can be nonsensical or seem strange, and that's okay. Don't let the analytical side in you filter or edit the experience. This is part of what makes ketamine journeys so special: The critical part of you goes offline.

Keep this experience as a lesson to take with you. Ketamine journeys help us relearn what it's like to live with awe, joy, presence, and childlike wonder. This helps to explain why so many clients report enhanced creativity after their sessions.

Later, you can come back to the "What it's telling me" column—immediately after the medicine wears off and/or in the days that follow. There will be some experiences that are easy to make sense of, and they'll come to you immediately. For other experiences, you may need to dialogue with your therapist in the *Integration* session to fully understand the meaning.

You also don't have to make sense of every single thing you experienced; the experiences that felt the most profound are usually the ones that are truly communicating something to you. In Ketamine-Assisted Psychotherapy, we believe that the places you go, emotional energies you experience, and loved ones who visit are so much more than "side effects" to be discarded. The medicine simply allows for and amplifies these messages to rise up into your conscious awareness. It helps to make the unconscious conscious, and can allow for integration of parts of yourself that had been warring, silent, dormant, or repressed—leading to wholeness or individuation.

1. Post-Journey Journal

EXPLORATION SESSION 1

The most important/overall message I received from my journey today was

And I can heed this message in the ordinary world of my waking life by

In my Integration session, I'd like to discuss or make sense of

WHAT I EXPERIENCED	WHAT IT MEANS

WHAT I EXPERIENCED	WHAT IT MEANS

Repeat the above for sessions 2 through 6.

2. At-Home Integration Activities

Here are some suggested activities when you get home:

- Light exercise or yoga. While ketamine tends to help people "leave" their physical body in their *Exploration* sessions, it also tends to help people feel reinvigorated upon return.

- Avoid all screens, e-mail, and work. Set your phone and e-mail to "Do Not Disturb."

- Avoid negative media.

  Consider: How would my life be better if I were exposed to less negative media pollution? Allow this time to be an experiment to see what that feels like. Discuss the results of your experiment in your *Integration* session.

- Eat healthy, nourishing meals (nothing out of the ordinary).

  When possible, consider meals that are unprocessed, plant-based, and free of added sugars. Sugar production and meat consumption are both linked to deforestation and global warming. They also tend to cause inflammation in the brain, which makes mental illness worse.

  Many people say that this type of diet can enhance their experience.

  Since this work tends to connect people with the earth and all living beings, how does this diet help care for the earth?

- Listen to relaxing music.

- Practice meditation, mindfulness, or other relaxation techniques.

- Use breath to relax or process emotions.

- Write or draw in a journal to capture thoughts, emotions, and memories that have gravitational pull or are otherwise worth recording.

- Take a walk or spend time in nature.

- Talk with supportive friends or family.

  This is not the time for stressful conversations, so save deeper conflict resolution for the day after. It can be helpful to discuss this in your *Integration* session. Many Field Trip patients find that they are better able to resolve conflict during or after their journey with us.

  Ketamine is a mild empathogen, so it tends to open people up.

The journey of Ketamine-Assisted Psychotherapy is both highly personal and nonlinear. The way you will grow and heal through your *Exploration* and *Integration* sessions depends on where you are and your personal goals. Like any psychotherapy session, it's hard to tell you exactly what you're going to talk about in session two versus session five. Our best advice to you is to stay present, stay open, go deeper, and take everything as it comes.

3. Additional Integration Exercises

We've included additional tools that many clients find helpful to incorporate throughout their journey. You are welcome to use one or all three of the tools at any point throughout your journey.

- **Going Deeper: The Unconscious, The Ego-Self Axis, and The Archetypes**

  This is a Jungian depth psychology technique that's helpful for people using KAP for deep, spiritual work.

- **Write Your Own Story: The Hero's Journey**

  This is a narrative therapy technique based on Joseph Campbell's Hero's Journey that's helpful for people feeling stuck or who need to create momentum in their life.

- **Thoughts, Behavior, and Daily ACES**

  This is a cognitive behavioral therapy technique that can help maximize, maintain, and extend the mood-boosting effects of Ketamine-Assisted Psychotherapy. For more information, see page 165.

GOING DEEPER: THE UNCONSCIOUS, THE EGO-SELF AXIS, AND THE ARCHETYPES

Ketamine-Assisted Psychotherapy is unique because it helps people dive below the level of the conscious mind—which is essential to true, root-cause-oriented healing. As you learned in Chapter 3, Jung believed the personal unconscious, shaped by personal experience, lies beneath the conscious mind. Underneath the personal unconscious lies the *collective* unconscious, which is inherited and contains information common to all human beings. Our deepest human instincts live at this level.

While some scientists used to scoff at the idea of a transpersonal collective unconscious, recent animal research has proven that fears can be inherited. Thus, science now provides at least some sort of validation for the "mystical" collective unconscious. Since Ketamine-Assisted Psychotherapy is a bio-psycho-social-spiritual approach, we don't shun the spiritual. Rather, we incorporate it into whole-person healing.

LEVEL 1: Conscious

LEVEL 2: Personal Unconscious

LEVEL 3: Collective Unconscious

Clients often report repressed or forgotten memories resurfacing in their *Exploration* sessions, which, of course, is an example of how ketamine provides direct access to the personal unconscious. In medium- and high-dose ketamine sessions, clients sometimes report experiences that don't originate from their own life history but feel highly significant. Many clients have the sensibility that these experiences are unearthed from the collective unconscious, that they are not just meaningless dreams or meanderings. Just hold this basic understanding of conscious, personal unconscious, and collective unconscious through your healing journey, because it proves to be a helpful framework for making sense of what is unearthed during your *Exploration* sessions.

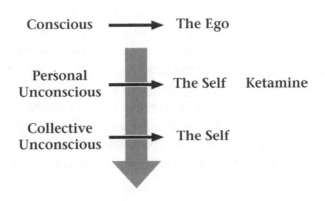

Now let's look at how the ego and the Self relate to the conscious and unconscious. The ego is most active at the level of the conscious, whereas the Self resides primarily in the unconscious. As a medicine, ketamine acts as a highly effective downward catalyst that helps you access material from the personal and collective unconscious quickly and deeply.

When you're born, you're in alignment with the Self (spelled with a capital *S*). As a baby, you don't understand the separateness between you, your caretakers, and the rest of the world. Psychologically, the Self is associated with wholeness or the unity of the personality. It has been called the "God within us" or your "highest self." Some spiritual traditions would call this the original nature of the "uncarved block," before life slices and dices its way to separateness. The Self is inherently whole and complete.

As you develop, the ego begins to emerge. You realize that you are separate from your caretakers and other beings. The ego's division between "you" and "them" can help you to be successful in our material world as you fight for your own needs. If your life has been filled with stability, support, and love, then the ego-Self axis remains intact. This is especially true for adults who have an ongoing spiritual practice or who have done deep work in psychotherapy or using other healing modalities. These entities coexist in relationship with each other.

But for many people in the modern world, trauma, instability, meaninglessness, materialism, and loneliness lead to the weakening or destruction of the ego-Self axis. Overidentification with the ego can result, which leads to existential depression and anxiety. Without service or connectedness, there is no meaning. There is only fighting for what serves *me*. There can be grandiosity, narcissism, or selfishness associated with a weakened or severed ego-Self axis.

Our goal is not to annihilate the ego and be totally aligned with Self. However, we also don't want to ignore Self and identify solely with ego. The ego, which is aligned with the conscious mind, is an important part of ourselves. But it's just the tip of the iceberg of the totality of who we are. Before Ketamine-Assisted Psychotherapy, we tend to see that most people are overidentified with ego with fleeting or forgotten experiences of the Self.

Since ketamine turns the ego down or off, your *Exploration* sessions remind you of how it feels to be aligned with the Self: connected, like a single point of consciousness, like "all is one," or like you are pure love. With the *Integration* sessions, there is a sense memory of this experience that becomes crystalized, and this becomes a reference point you can carry with you in your waking life.

In this diagram, you'll see the way the ego and the Self can coexist and are connected via the ego-Self axis. The restitution of this axis is one of the primary goals of Ketamine-Assisted Psychotherapy. When you consider how you will take your special message from an *Exploration* session into your waking life, you're rebuilding the ego-Self axis. We hope this journey leaves you more whole.

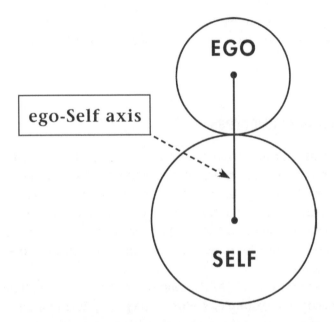

Here are some reflection questions that can help you integrate and rebuild a healthy ego-Self axis.

My ego looks or sounds like . . .

I know I am overidentified with my ego when I . . .

The Self looks or sounds like . . .

I know I am having an experience aligned with the Self when I . . .

Previously, I thought the relationship between the ego and the Self was . . .

My *Exploration* sessions are helping to restore the ego-Self axis by . . .

If the ego could say something to the Self, it would probably say . . .

If the Self could say something to the ego, it would probably say . . .

One thing I can do to preserve the relationship between the ego and the Self is . . .

In your *Exploration* sessions, have any important memories, lessons, or experiences surfaced from the level of the personal unconscious? If so, what are the most profound ones?

WORKING WITH ARCHETYPES

Now let's turn our attention to the archetypes. Many clients will have an experience of one or more of the archetypes in their *Exploration* sessions. Archetypes are "the forms which the instincts assume" and "unfiltered psychic experience." They surface from the level of the collective unconscious, but upon integration they can rise up to the level of the conscious. We've found working with archetypes can also help restore a healthy ego-Self axis and make people feel more whole.

Archetypes that surface in *Exploration* sessions tend to be aligned with a client's timely needs. For example, seeing a magician during a ketamine journey may be saying to a client who has forgotten his or her self-worth, "You have the power within you to make your dreams come true." In *Integration* sessions, you and your therapist may discuss what you can do in your ordinary, waking life to be more powerful, and why the magician appeared to you at this time. If you can identify the archetypes within yourself during integration, you will probably be able to identify dominant archetypes within others. Even businesses and brands have dominant archetypes, so you may even become more aware of why you're drawn to a certain product or type of experience.

This lens helps us move away from a pathology-based, black-or-white way of thinking so we can create a space for you to hold all of your parts. Instead of labeling yourself as too needy or too domineering, you can acknowledge that it's an archetype, or part, within you that is common to all people. Many people doing this work say it helps them to be gentler toward themselves, because you don't have to be "all good," nor are you "all bad." When you become aware of the parts within you, you can strive for greater balance.

Here are the 12 archetypes. At any point during integration, you may wish to answer the questions related to each archetype—especially when an archetype surfaces in a ketamine journey. As you read through these 12 archetypes, you may be able to quickly identify your most dominant archetype as well as ones that may need to speak up. It's not uncommon for clients to report that before Ketamine-Assisted Psychotherapy, the dominant archetype functioned like a dictator making all the decisions. Through the journey of Ketamine-Assisted Psychotherapy, it begins to feel like a democracy where all the archetypes have a seat at the table of your life.

1. The Innocent

Motto: "Free to be you and me."
Core desire: to get to paradise
Goal: to be happy
Greatest fear: to be punished for doing something bad or wrong
Strategy: to do things right
Weakness: boring for all their naive innocence
Talent: faith, optimism
Also known as: the utopian, the traditionalist, the naïf, the mystic, the saint, the romantic, the dreamer

Do you have a name for this part of you?

What does this archetype want?

How does this archetype help you in your life?

Where did this archetype come from?

When do you know this archetype is running the show in your life?

Does this archetype need to be more or less active?

What do you love about this part of you?

How dominant or disowned is this archetype?

What would you say to this archetype?

What would this archetype say to you?

Does this archetype have anything to say to other parts of you?

2. The Orphan or Regular Guy/Gal

Motto: "All people are created equal."
Core desire: connecting with others
Goal: to belong
Greatest fear: to be left out or to stand out from the crowd
Strategy: develop ordinary, solid virtues; be down to earth; the common touch
Weakness: losing one's own self in an effort to blend in or for the sake of superficial relationships
Talent: realism, empathy, lack of pretense
Also known as: the good old boy, the everyman, the person next door, the realist, the working stiff, the solid citizen, the good neighbor, the silent majority

Do you have a name for this part of you?

What does this archetype want?

How does this archetype help you in your life?

Where did this archetype come from?

When do you know this archetype is running the show in your life?

Does this archetype need to be more or less active?

What do you love about this part of you?

How dominant or disowned is this archetype?

What would you say to this archetype?

What would this archetype say to you?

Does this archetype have anything to say to other parts of you?

3. The Hero

Motto: "Where there's a will, there's a way."
Core desire: to prove one's worth through courageous acts
Goal: expert mastery in a way that improves the world
Greatest fear: weakness, vulnerability, being a "chicken"
Strategy: to be as strong and competent as possible
Weakness: arrogance, always needing another battle to fight
Talent: competence, courage
Also known as: the warrior, the crusader, the rescuer, the superhero, the soldier, the dragon slayer, the winner, the team player

Do you have a name for this part of you?

What does this archetype want?

How does this archetype help you in your life?

Where did this archetype come from?

When do you know this archetype is running the show in your life?

Does this archetype need to be more or less active?

What do you love about this part of you?

How dominant or disowned is this archetype?

What would you say to this archetype?

What would this archetype say to you?

Does this archetype have anything to say to other parts of you?

4. The Caregiver

Motto: "Love your neighbor as yourself."
Core desire: to protect and care for others
Goal: to help others
Greatest fear: selfishness and ingratitude
Strategy: doing things for others

Weakness: martyrdom and being exploited
Talent: compassion, generosity
Also known as: the saint, the altruist, the parent, the helper, the supporter

Do you have a name for this part of you?

What does this archetype want?

How does this archetype help you in your life?

Where did this archetype come from?

When do you know this archetype is running the show in your life?

Does this archetype need to be more or less active?

What do you love about this part of you?

How dominant or disowned is this archetype?

What would you say to this archetype?

What would this archetype say to you?

Does this archetype have anything to say to other parts of you?

5. The Explorer

Motto: "Don't fence me in."
Core desire: the freedom to find out who they are through exploring the world
Goal: to experience a better, more authentic, more fulfilling life
Biggest fear: getting trapped, conformity, inner emptiness
Strategy: journey, seeking out and experiencing new things, escape
from boredom
Weakness: aimless wandering, becoming a misfit
Talent: autonomy, ambition, being true to one's soul
Also known as: the seeker, the iconoclast, the wanderer, the individualist,
the pilgrim

Do you have a name for this part of you?

What does this archetype want?

How does this archetype help you in your life?

Where did this archetype come from?

When do you know this archetype is running the show in your life?

Does this archetype need to be more or less active?

What do you love about this part of you?

How dominant or disowned is this archetype?

What would you say to this archetype?

What would this archetype say to you?

Does this archetype have anything to say to other parts of you?

6. The Rebel

Motto: "Rules are made to be broken."
Core desire: revenge or revolution
Goal: to overturn what isn't working
Greatest fear: to be powerless or ineffectual
Strategy: disrupt, destroy, shock
Weakness: crossing over to the dark side, crime
Talent: outrageousness, radical freedom
Also known as: the rebel, the revolutionary, the wild man, the misfit, the iconoclast

Do you have a name for this part of you?

What does this archetype want?

How does this archetype help you in your life?

Where did this archetype come from?

When do you know this archetype is running the show in your life?

Does this archetype need to be more or less active?

What do you love about this part of you?

How dominant or disowned is this archetype?

What would you say to this archetype?

What would this archetype say to you?

Does this archetype have anything to say to other parts of you?

7. The Lover

Motto: "You're the only one."
Core desire: intimacy and experience
Goal: being in a relationship with the people, work, and surroundings they love
Greatest fear: being alone, a wallflower, unwanted, unloved
Strategy: to become more and more physically and emotionally attractive
Weakness: outward-directed desire to please others at the risk of losing their own identity
Talent: passion, gratitude, appreciation, commitment
Also known as: the partner, the friend, the intimate, the enthusiast, the sensualist, the spouse, the team builder

Do you have a name for this part of you?

What does this archetype want?

How does this archetype help you in your life?

Where did this archetype come from?

When do you know this archetype is running the show in your life?

Does this archetype need to be more or less active?

What do you love about this part of you?

How dominant or disowned is this archetype?

What would you say to this archetype?

What would this archetype say to you?

Does this archetype have anything to say to other parts of you?

8. The Creator

Motto: "If you can imagine it, it can be done."
Core desire: to create things of enduring value
Goal: to realize a vision
Greatest fear: mediocre vision or execution
Strategy: develop artistic control and skill
Task: to create culture, express own vision
Weakness: perfectionism, bad solutions
Talent: creativity, imagination
Also known as: the artist, the inventor, the innovator, the musician, the writer, the dreamer

Do you have a name for this part of you?

What does this archetype want?

How does this archetype help you in your life?

Where did this archetype come from?

When do you know this archetype is running the show in your life?

Does this archetype need to be more or less active?

What do you love about this part of you?

How dominant or disowned is this archetype?

What would you say to this archetype?

What would this archetype say to you?

Does this archetype have anything to say to other parts of you?

9. The Jester

Motto: "You only live once."
Core desire: to live in the moment with full enjoyment
Goal: to have a great time and lighten up the world
Greatest fear: being bored or boring others
Strategy: play, make jokes, be funny
Weakness: frivolity, wasting time
Talent: joy
Also known as: the fool, the trickster, the joker, the practical joker, the comedian

Do you have a name for this part of you?

What does this archetype want?

How does this archetype help you in your life?

Where did this archetype come from?

When do you know this archetype is running the show in your life?

Does this archetype need to be more or less active?

What do you love about this part of you?

How dominant or disowned is this archetype?

What would you say to this archetype?

What would this archetype say to you?

Does this archetype have anything to say to other parts of you?

10. The Sage

Motto: "The truth will set you free."
Core desire: to find the truth
Goal: to use intelligence and analysis to understand the world
Biggest fear: being duped or misled; ignorance

Strategy: seeking out information and knowledge; self-reflection and understanding thought processes
Weakness: can study details forever and never act
Talent: wisdom, intelligence
Also known as: the expert, the scholar, the detective, the adviser, the thinker, the philosopher, the academic, the researcher, the planner, the professional, the mentor, the teacher, the contemplative

Do you have a name for this part of you?

What does this archetype want?

How does this archetype help you in your life?

Where did this archetype come from?

When do you know this archetype is running the show in your life?

Does this archetype need to be more or less active?

What do you love about this part of you?

How dominant or disowned is this archetype?

What would you say to this archetype?

What would this archetype say to you?

Does this archetype have anything to say to other parts of you?

11. The Magician

Motto: "I make things happen."
Core desire: understanding the fundamental laws of the universe
Goal: to make dreams come true
Greatest fear: unintended negative consequences
Strategy: develop a vision and live by it
Weakness: becoming manipulative
Talent: finding win-win solutions

Also known as: the visionary, the catalyst, the inventor, the charismatic leader, the shaman, the healer, the medicine man

Do you have a name for this part of you?

What does this archetype want?

How does this archetype help you in your life?

Where did this archetype come from?

When do you know this archetype is running the show in your life?

Does this archetype need to be more or less active?

What do you love about this part of you?

How dominant or disowned is this archetype?

What would you say to this archetype?

What would this archetype say to you?

Does this archetype have anything to say to other parts of you?

12. The Ruler

Motto: "Power isn't everything, it's the only thing."
Core desire: control
Goal: create a prosperous, successful family or community
Strategy: exercise power
Greatest fear: chaos, being overthrown
Weakness: being authoritarian, unable to delegate
Talent: responsibility, leadership
Also known as: the boss, the leader, the aristocrat, the king, the queen, the politician, the role model, the manager, the administrator

Do you have a name for this part of you?

What does this archetype want?

How does this archetype help you in your life?

Where did this archetype come from?

When do you know this archetype is running the show in your life?

Does this archetype need to be more or less active?

What do you love about this part of you?

How dominant or disowned is this archetype?

What would you say to this archetype?

What would this archetype say to you?

Does this archetype have anything to say to other parts of you?

WRITE YOUR OWN STORY: THE HERO'S JOURNEY

Whether you already know it or not, you're already quite familiar with the hero's journey. If you've watched a Disney film like *Beauty and the Beast,* you know the basic structure of the fairy tale and can easily recognize its hero. *The Wizard of Oz* has Dorothy; *Harry Potter and the Sorcerer's Stone* has Harry; *The Matrix* has Neo. And your story, of course, has *you.*

The hero's journey is based on Professor Joseph Campbell's 1949 book *The Hero with a Thousand Faces.* In his research for the book, Campbell studied religious figures, myths, fairy tales, and literary classics that have shaped our world. While religious or spiritual beliefs are not required to go on a hero's journey, they are also not excluded—if a certain belief system resonates with you. Jung would say that the reason archetypes have shown up across cultures for thousands of years is because they have always been in the collective unconscious.

In a wildly popular PBS documentary about the hero's journey, Campbell explained that the process requires the hero to undergo a symbolic "death and resurrection . . . and that is the basic motif of the hero's journey: leaving one condition, finding the source of life to bring you forth in a richer, more mature, or 'other' condition."

Consider these three simple questions as they relate to your journey of Ketamine-Assisted Psychotherapy.

1. The condition or world I'm leaving behind is _____ .
2. The "source of life" I'm finding is _____ .
3. Back in the ordinary world, I'd like to return in a condition marked by

   _____ .

Let's examine the hero's journey fully. The story begins with the protagonist in an ordinary world. Dorothy is in Kansas, Harry lives in the cupboard under the stairs at 4 Privet Drive, and you spend most of your time here in this ordinary world on planet Earth.

Then, the hero is called to leave this world and enter a magical world. Harry departs for the magical world on the Hogwarts Express from platform 9¾. In *The Matrix*, Neo is presented with a choice: "You take the blue pill . . . the story ends, you wake up in your bed, and believe whatever you want to believe. You take the red pill . . . you stay in Wonderland, and I show you how deep the rabbit hole goes." You have embarked on a "magical" ketamine journey deep into the unconscious where other worlds, whole-person healing, and even spiritual enlightenment is possible.

Did you hesitate before starting this journey—or at some point along the way? If so, just know that resistance is part of the hero's journey, too. All heroes at some point or another have said to themselves, *Why me?* But if you're stuck in the dull, gray world that is a hallmark of depression, perhaps it's time to go to Oz and awaken to the Technicolor spectrum of your rich and beautiful life.

The hero's journey that is Ketamine-Assisted Psychotherapy will be one of many hero's journeys you will embark on in your life. A positive experience like following your true calling is a hero's journey. Moving, divorce, loss, and other transitions can be part of a hero's journey, too. A hero's journey is not black or white—and it's not finite.

There are 12 stages in the hero's journey. Some journeys may include all 12 stages in order, while others may incorporate only some of the stages. You might have already begun to recognize the many hero's journeys you've previously been on. In taking the medicine in your *Exploration* sessions, you have taken the proverbial red pill and are learning something new about yourself.

You now have a basic understanding of the archetypes. Besides the hero, there is also the sage. The sage in *Star Wars* is Obi-Wan Kenobi. Harry Potter's sage is Dumbledore. Who will be the sage in your story—or how you will learn to listen to the sage within you? In the lexicon of psychedelic-assisted psychotherapy, the sage may be part of your "inner healing intelligence" or "inner therapist."

Is there one particular fairy tale or movie that you can think of that resonated with you in a deep way? The wonderful thing about fairy tales and stories is that because we're watching a story about someone else, it slides past the self-protecting defenses of the ego. The ego isn't confronted and is free to project onto the characters. Information from the unconscious can rise up without a filter—just as it does in your *Exploration* sessions. The way we tend to be affected by archetypal characters and feel so deeply is because these stories reflect parts of ourselves, whether those parts are integrated or disowned.

Have you ever rooted for the hero but simultaneously felt for the villain? That's because we all have to learn how to hold space for our whole selves, and we all have parts that could be thought of as both hero and villain. Even Luke Skywalker had to acknowledge the similarities between his father, Darth Vader, and himself. This work can help us put an end to a common defense mechanism called splitting—a type of black-or-white thinking in which an idea, person, or group is perceived as either all good or all bad. You can probably see the way splitting is even becoming a more common practice in our increasingly polarized world. Conversely, could this type of work help people to be a beacon of peace?

Through the hero's journey, you may learn how to identify and integrate your "shadow." When you're unaware of your shadow, it can take over you—like it did for Anakin Skywalker when he became Darth Vader. If you can confront it and integrate it, you can identify it and not allow it to take over. As Jung said: "This meeting with oneself is, at first, the meeting with one's own shadow. The shadow is a tight passage, a narrow door, whose painful constriction no one is spared who goes down to the deep well. But one must learn to know oneself in order to know who one is."

Unlike other psychotherapy treatments where the primary goal is to seek symptom elimination, our goal is *individuation*. Other treatments want to eradicate the parts of you that are deemed "bad" or pathological. We want to facilitate peace between the parts of you. Jung said: "Individuation means becoming 'individual,' and in so far as 'individuality' embraces our innermost, last, and incomparable uniqueness, it also implies becoming one's own self. We could therefore translate individuation as 'coming to selfhood.'"

I suspect coming "to selfhood" will help you lead a richer and more fulfilling life—which is, of course, one of the most powerful antidotes to depression, anxiety, PTSD, addiction, or the journey we call being human. I wonder how it can help you to love yourself more and become unstuck in your life.

The hero's journey is a powerful tool that can help you do deep and transformative work—and discover the true roots of depression, anxiety, malaise, or a general feeling of being stuck. By moving through this journey, you will return to the ordinary world with the elixir that will change you in profound ways.

Consider the visual representation of the hero's journey below. Notice the threshold between the ordinary world and the special world. The first time you took the medicine, you crossed the first threshold and entered into "the special world" of the ketamine journey.

When the medicine wears off, it's time for reentry into the "ordinary world." You may cross this threshold several times if you're doing multiple *Exploration* sessions, as most clients do. Making sense of what you experienced will help you integrate lessons into your everyday life. You'll understand what "elixir" you are bringing back with you. You could also apply the hero's journey to a significant life issue like addiction or loss, with Ketamine-Assisted Psychotherapy being a part of that journey. Only you know how rich your story is. While others can provide guidance, only you can write your story.

While I don't know what elixir you'll come back with, I do know that clients tend to find whatever elixir they need most for true, complete healing. It can be a newfound motivation to live a full life, a spiritual lesson to find the awe and wonder in daily life, or perhaps the hope you've been yearning to find for years. We all have an inner healing intelligence within. No doctor needs to give that to you, because, like Dorothy did with the ruby slippers, you will eventually realize that you had what you needed within you this whole time.

Here is your chance to write your story based on the 12 stages of the hero's journey. Remember: You don't necessarily have to come up with something for each step. Read each step and see what comes forth. Consider this exercise a template to deepen your work. It can be helpful to write this in the third person. By doing so, you can integrate different parts of yourself that you encounter through your journey and move toward wholeness.

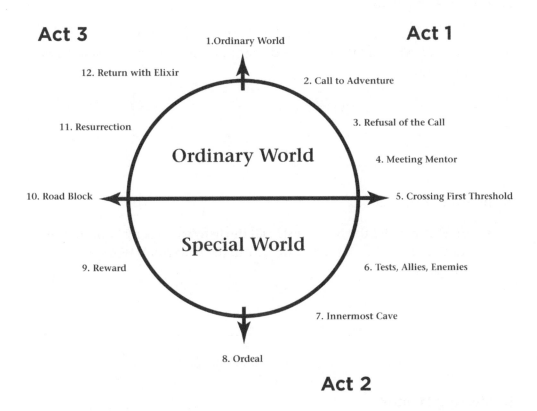

Act 3

Act 1

1. Ordinary World

12. Return with Elixir

2. Call to Adventure

11. Resurrection

3. Refusal of the Call

4. Meeting Mentor

Ordinary World

10. Road Block

5. Crossing First Threshold

Special World

9. Reward

6. Tests, Allies, Enemies

7. Innermost Cave

8. Ordeal

Act 2

ACT 1: ORDINARY WORLD

1. Ordinary World

- How would you describe your "ordinary world" before the hero (i.e., you) embarked on the journey—whether it was Ketamine-Assisted Psychotherapy itself or another journey in your life? What did this world look and feel like for the hero?

_____

_____

_____

2. Call to Adventure

- When did the hero hear the call to do this deep work and change his/her life? What did the call sound like? In what form was it delivered to the hero?

_____

_____

_____

3. Refusal of the Call

- In what way did the hero resist? Did the hero try to deny or minimize the importance of doing this work? Did the hero think _Why me_ at any point?

_____

_____

_____

4. Meeting Mentor

- Who was the mentor or mentors the hero met before embarking on this journey? How would you describe this meeting? Why was this meeting significant?

_____

_____

_____

ACT 2: SPECIAL WORLD

5. Crossing the First Threshold

- What was the threshold into the special world? Once the hero committed to this journey, how did he or she feel? How did the hero feel knowing that this was the first step in creating change?

_____

_____

_____

6. Tests, Allies, Enemies

- How was the hero tested and able to make it through the trials? Who were the hero's allies? Who were the enemies? How did the hero recognize who the allies and enemies were? How did the hero respond?

_____

_____

_____

7. Innermost Cave

- Did any old or unresolved wounds resurface here—in the place where the hero prepared for deep change and inner work? Did the hero let go of mindsets, beliefs, or limiting beliefs that needed to be changed?

_____

_____

_____

8. Ordeal

- Did the hero reach a rock bottom? If so, what did that feel like? How did the hero move through the pain, sadness, or loneliness? Why did the hero need to feel those in order to change?

_____

_____

_____

9. Reward

- After the hero faced all of these challenges, how was he or she rewarded? What changed for the hero? How did the hero feel? What were the internal and external rewards the hero received? How did the rewards help the hero to keep going?

_____

_____

_____

ACT 3: BACK IN THE ORDINARY WORLD

10. The Road Back

- As the hero rededicated him or herself to change, did the hero reflect on this journey? Why was every step essential on this journey? How did that feel? What has changed at this point in the journey?

_____

_____

_____

11. Resurrection

- As the hero's journey came to an end, were there any final attempts to change in the ordinary world? How did the hero gain self-mastery? How did some part of the hero die so that he or she could be reborn as the highest self? Did the hero change the way he or she felt about him or herself?

_____

_____

_____

12. Return with Elixir

- The hero is now home. He or she has had time to reflect upon the journey. What is the elixir that the hero now has? How is this changing the hero's life? What does this feel like? How will you share this elixir with the world? If Act I was aligned with the ego and Act II was aligned with the Self, how does the elixir help the hero to restore the relationship between the ego and the Self? How is the hero's life here in the ordinary world helping him or her integrate what he or she has learned? How will the hero know to embark upon another journey?

_____

_____

_____

To complement these depth-oriented tools, the following section will help you incorporate cognitive behavioral therapy (CBT) tools, too. At first, Jungian-based analytical and depth psychology and cognitive behavioral therapy may seem like two opposing models that can't possibly fit together. But in many ways, changing what you do in "the ordinary world" is a way of heeding the messages you receive in the "special world." If you don't do anything differently in the ordinary world, then you have not yet fulfilled your hero's journey. It would be like Dorothy waking up and saying to herself, "Well, that was weird," and going about her day. When she's back in Kansas, you have a sense that her heart is filled with love and appreciates the people in her life even more. It may also be helpful to complete A and understand the ego-Self axis, because the "elixir of life" you'll bring back will mean you'll want to achieve, connect, enjoy, and preserve the ego-Self axis on a daily basis.

THOUGHTS, BEHAVIOR, AND DAILY ACES

To complement the deep work and to help you maintain the afterglow associated with Ketamine-Assisted Psychotherapy, it's time to change your thoughts and your actions—the essence of cognitive behavioral therapy (CBT). As you know, ketamine lifts neurotransmitters and enhances neurogenesis. That improvement makes this an ideal time to create new, healthy ways of thinking and acting in the world—which will make the improvements you're experiencing last longer.

Let's first take a look at how the *cognitive* part of cognitive behavioral therapy changes you. By changing the way you think, you change what you do. By changing what you do, you change the way you feel. The end result: an improvement in your mood.

THOUGHTS ➡ BEHAVIOR ➡ FEELING = MOOD IMPROVEMENT

For example, a client in Ketamine-Assisted Psychotherapy realizes that his relationship anxiety stems from the abandonment and neglect he experienced in his childhood. In addition to the deep reprocessing that occurs in *Exploration* and *Integration* sessions, his therapist helps him to change pitfall thought patterns like pessimistic and catastrophic thinking (e.g., *She's going to leave at some point anyway. Everyone does.*). By eliciting contrary evidence to this irrational fear (e.g., *I do have several people in my life who have stuck by me no matter what.*), he eventually notices that his actions in relationships begin to change (e.g., not texting his new girlfriend multiple times within an hour if he doesn't hear back from her). He begins to feel more peaceful in his daily life, and the mood lift from Ketamine-Assisted Psychotherapy lasts longer. It has been a year, and he notices his perspective shift has led to a permanent improvement in mood. Should he hit a bump in the road, he is more than willing to return for a maintenance *Exploration* session should he need it.

On the other hand, the *behavioral* part of cognitive behavioral therapy flows in the opposite direction: By changing what you *do*, you can change how you think. This improves the way you feel.

BEHAVIOR ➡ THOUGHTS ➡ FEELING = MOOD IMPROVEMENT

For example, a woman experiencing depression has profound aha moments in her *Exploration* and *Integration* sessions. She is also noticing a profound improvement in her mood, energy, hunger, and sleep patterns. The woman and her therapist take advantage of this lift by making sure she does one thing every day that gives her a sense of achievement. This, like ketamine itself, lifts dopamine. There is a synergistic benefit to combining the medicine with this behavioral tool.

This leads to her feeling more hopeful and reduces pitfall thought patterns like paralysis by analysis (e.g., *I just can't stop thinking about all the disappointing events in my life. It's hard to even focus on work.*). Without these limiting beliefs, she feels hopeful and confident. She eventually realizes that her way of being can be changed—if she leads with action. Ketamine's empathogenic effects provide a deep compassion for self and others, which works synergistically with these changes in her behavior. The lift from Ketamine-Assisted Psychotherapy is robust, and she does not need to return for a maintenance *Exploration* session for five months. She finds this rhythm to be highly effective for her.

Ketamine-Assisted Psychotherapy takes advantage of this unique window of opportunity. Instead of just changing thoughts/feelings or behavior, Ketamine-Assisted Psychotherapy acknowledges that there is a bidirectional relationship between thoughts/feelings and behavior—but takes it a step further. Unlike traditional medication for depression and anxiety, *Exploration* sessions lead to deep and profound insights. This too improves mood, which then changes how a client thinks, feels, and acts—and vice versa. The insights that follow tend to be deeper, which catalyzes even more change.

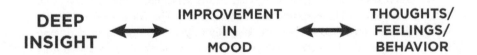

DEEP INSIGHT ⬅➡ IMPROVEMENT IN MOOD ⬅➡ THOUGHTS/ FEELINGS/ BEHAVIOR

Now that you understand the basic philosophy of how we combine Ketamine-Assisted Psychotherapy with cognitive behavioral therapy, it's time to turn our attention to the way *you* think and act. The *C* in CBT stands for *cognitive*. Read through the seven pitfall thought patterns. As you do, take note of the top three pitfall thought patterns that have held you back the most, and then complete the following steps.

7 Pitfall Thought Patterns, by Dr. Mike Dow

1. **Paralysis-analysis:** This type of thinking involves stewing and ruminating in anxious thoughts, preventing productive action from occurring. For example: *I wonder why Harmony got that account and not me. Does my boss like her better than me? I wonder if it's because of that mistake I made last month on that account. My boss said he wasn't mad, but maybe he was and just didn't want to tell me. He did give me a sort of funny look this morning. I'm so behind on this project, but I just can't stop thinking about this. I'm freaking out . . .*

2. **Permanence:** This type of thinking falsely assumes that just because something is a problem now, it will always be a problem. Mood-congruent recall in the brain lights up negative memories in the brain, creating the illusion that you've always been stressed and therefore will always be stressed in the future. For example: *Dealing with my dad's health problems is so hard, and it feels like it's never going to end. My life is hard, and it feels like it's always been this way. This dark cloud isn't going to pass.*

3. **Personalization:** This type of thinking places the blame entirely on yourself for something not going your way. The error here is that there are multiple people as well as circumstances that are involved in unfavorable outcomes. Perhaps there are some things you'd like to change, but it's rarely *entirely* your fault, just as it's rarely *entirely* the other person's fault. For example: *My divorce was my fault. It happened because I'm unlovable. I must not be capable of being in a relationship. I'm weak.*

4. **Pervasiveness:** This type of thinking allows something that is affecting one area of your life to spread to all areas of your life. For example: *What a stressful day! I can't deal with one more person. I'm going to skip yoga and get out of my dinner plans. I'd rather just sit alone by myself in front of the TV and eat pizza.*

5. **Pessimistic:** This type of thinking considers the worst-case, catastrophic scenario. It dwells in the possible—not the probable. For example: *If I don't get my anxiety under control, I'll probably start having panic attacks several times a day. How will I ever be able to work if I have uncontrollable panic attacks? If I started having one when I'm driving, I'd crash my car and kill someone. Maybe I'll get sent to prison. How would I ever live with that guilt?*

6. **Polarized:** This type of thinking has a binary, black-or-white pattern. The words *always* or *never* are frequently found in this type of thought pattern. For example: *I've always had sleeping problems. If my insomnia isn't 100 percent better, then I've failed. There are two types of people: good sleepers and insomniacs. I'm the latter.*

7. **Psychic:** This type of thinking expects people around us to read our minds without us verbalizing what we need. It can also mean falsely assuming we know what someone else is thinking even when they haven't verbalized their opinion. For example: *My friends aren't helping me. Can't they see I'm struggling? They haven't even asked me how I'm doing tonight, and if you look at my face, you can see something's wrong. If they really knew me and cared about my well-being, they'd know this and would do something to help me feel better. I feel so alone.*

STEP 1: IDENTIFYING PITFALL THOUGHT PATTERNS

Now, note below the top three pitfall thought patterns that have held you back the most.

1.

2.

3.

Identifying your top pitfall thought patterns can help you to notice when they are floating into your conscious awareness.

STEP 2: CREATE A NONJUDGMENTAL CONTAINER ALIGNED WITH THE SELF

Now that you've had an experience of being aligned with the Self during ketamine journeys, you will probably find it easier to distance yourself from these—since they tend to originate in the ego. They aren't facts; they're information. Be the container that allows these negative thoughts to come and go. You can imagine yourself saying to these thoughts: "Hello, personalization that's coming from the ego. I see you. You're creating separateness and causing me to compare myself to others. Now that I've had an experience of oneness, I can simply allow you to float on by."

How has your *Exploration* session(s) helped you to create a nonjudgmental container for pitfall thought patterns? In what ways are you noticing yourself being less affected by them?

STEP 3: TALKING BACK TO PITFALL THOUGHT PATTERNS

Go back to your top three pitfall thought patterns. Imagine that you're now going to talk back to them by eliciting the contrary evidence, proving them wrong. For many people, it can feel like this talking back is originating from the Self or your inner healing intelligence. People tend to leave Ketamine-Assisted Psychotherapy feeling more confident and hopeful. With the profound improvement in mood, you may even realize how much of your negative thoughts and feelings were actually your depression or anxiety—not you.

1. Pitfall Thought Pattern:
The contrary evidence that proves this pitfall thought pattern wrong is:

2. Pitfall Thought Pattern:
The contrary evidence that proves this pitfall thought pattern wrong is:

3. Pitfall Thought Pattern:
The contrary evidence that proves this pitfall thought pattern wrong is:

Now it's time to turn our attention to the *B* in CBT: *behavioral*. Many clients say that after an *Exploration* session, they are suddenly able to do things that felt impossible before. It's vital that you take advantage of this unique window of opportunity. If you're working your way through a month that includes multiple *Preparation*, *Exploration*, and *Integration* sessions, your therapist will help support you and provide accountability.

What a wonderful time to try on new ways of being in the world! Through your journey in Ketamine-Assisted Psychotherapy, we recommend adding ACES: achievement, closeness, enjoyment, and the Self. Add one activity each day that brings one of these four qualities to your life.

A: Achievement. Doing something that gives you a sense of productivity lifts dopamine, just like ketamine. What is something that fills you with a sense of achievement? How does this help you create a life filled with possibilities? If you saw a life filled with hope and light in your *Exploration* session, then doing something that brings you a sense of achievement is a way of manifesting this life—and, thus, bringing the special world of ketamine journeys and the ordinary world closer together.

C: Closeness. Interpersonal connection is vital to good mood. It's a tonic against mental illness and helps you boost serotonin and oxytocin. As you know, being lonely is associated with an overactive default mode network (DMN). Since ketamine turns the DMN down, doing something that helps you connect to others makes sure this DMN doesn't become overactive again.

E: Enjoyment. Doing something that brings you pleasure can lift neurotransmitters like dopamine and serotonin. What is a self-care activity you really enjoy doing? Can you bring the sense of childlike awe and wonder you rediscovered in your *Exploration* sessions to these activities? Does it help you find joy in the simplest of activities?

S: The Self. Anything spiritual like meditation, prayer, hypnosis, yoga, breath-work, or time in nature can help you make sure the ego-Self axis stays aligned. It can prevent the ego from becoming overactive and help you retain the mystical sense that "all is one" you may have received in your *Exploration* sessions. Like ketamine, self-care activities aligned with the Self can ensure the DMN doesn't become overactive.

In the table below, note the date. Then note one activity you did that brought you a sense of achievement, closeness, enjoyment, and the Self each day. Then note your overall mood that day on a scale of 1 to 10—with 10 being the best. This helps you do two things. First, it helps you notice the relationship between what you do and how you feel, creating a positive feedback loop. Second, you can identify when your mood is dipping more than a few points from where you were, which can be an indication that it's time to return for a maintenance *Exploration* session.

Date	Achievement	Closeness	Enjoyment	The Self	Mood: 1–10

Date	Achievement	Closeness	Enjoyment	The Self	Mood: 1–10

CHAPTER 13

THE KAP WORKBOOK: EXTENDING THE AFTERGLOW

You may never feel so good as you do coming away from your KAP experiences. We call it the "afterglow" period when life is light, tranquil, and filled with joyful wonder. You have a new sense of strength with being at ease in your body. You're much quicker to laugh or smile, while having an advanced ability to let negativity roll off your shoulders. There's no more stress or sadness, as your ability to grow and address difficulties has increased. It's like the feeling of falling in love, only this time you're falling in love with yourself. This afterglow lasts for days, weeks, even months—or perhaps the rest of your life.

Still, we recommend a few strategies that can extend this afterglow, maintain the feeling, and facilitate further growth into who you are becoming. Be sure to take full advantage of the tools that can help the afterglow last longer. Plus, you'll want to monitor yourself so you know when your defenses are weakened. You definitely don't want to ignore the signs and symptoms of losing ground. And there are some things, and people, you definitely want to avoid so that you can keep the afterglow . . . glowing.

PRACTICE MEDITATION

Developing a meditation practice is like having a superpower. It can calm your mind, enhance focus, and bring you back to center. Plus, meditating is probably the best way to extend the afterglow because you can evoke those ketamine-like feelings again, going back whenever you like. For those recovering from addictions, meditation becomes an invaluable tool if/when overwhelming thoughts and emotions begin to feel unmanageable. Meditation allows you to tune in to yourself and who you are becoming. So we highly recommend practicing daily meditation to extend the afterglow.

CONTINUE WITH THERAPY

This is not the time to stop going to your therapist. In fact, it's fertile ground to continue the growth process that KAP began. Plus, having regular time with your therapist will continue to percolate issues to the surface for you to learn from. Now you'll have enlightened awareness and confidence to build onto the foundations you've laid with KAP.

CONNECT WITH COMMUNITY

Something amazing happens on the journey when you find a community of like-minded individuals who support each other based on their own personal experiences. The alternative is to stay isolated, both in our head and logistically, which separates us from forming a healthy group of people seeking enrichment as well. People who connect with a community understand this, and people who haven't just don't.

When you find a group of people, whether in person or online, you'll find freedom to talk about the most esoteric or weird subjects that came up during your KAP regimen. You'll find an audience who can relate, and be equally amazed, and will love you for sharing. This vulnerability breeds internal strength. Besides, it's a win-win for everyone involved.

It's like veterans from the military who share a deep bond because of what they went through *together*. Imagine having that with others because of a shared love and respect for a very cool psychedelic experience. Having a community gives you people to turn to when times get hard, and helps you avoid reverting to old patterns of thought and behavior. Community strengthens what you've learned during integration and will keep the afterglow burning.

You can find psychedelic meetups, and you can use the Field Trip App, which can connect you with others.

AVOID ABUSING ALCOHOL, AND STREET DRUGS

Just because we've used ketamine to rewire your brain and behavior doesn't mean we condone turning to the party scene, with drugs and alcohol, to solve all your problems. It's quite the opposite. Alcohol is a depressant, and abusing it only makes matters worse and can undo much of the progress accomplished with KAP. While cannabis can be productive, it too can be abused to the point of derailing your progress. Nor should you go find a drug dealer and score some "Special K" on the street. It's unsafe, with unknown purity and potency. Plus, without medical supervision and integration guided by a licensed therapist, your trip can be in vain.

After going through KAP, you'll come out a different person—more stable, more enlightened, and more aware. To keep that afterglow lit, we recommend being good to yourself. The ketamine experience is meant to be a catalyst for change and to leave the problematic overuse of drugs and alcohol behind.

LEAN INTO PROGRESS

Now that you've opened your eyes to a whole new world of possibilities through KAP, the personal growth journey is just getting started. There are many ways to explore freedoms in thoughts and behaviors that benefit your overall well-being. Instead of thinking, *Well, I've done KAP and I'm better now*, lean into the here and now of what you can become. Your world can become even brighter, more interesting, more nuanced, and more textured and exciting. The more you do this personal growth work, the more happiness you will find. It's like the expression "Happiness resides not in experiencing new things, but in seeing the world through new eyes."

When you've found freedom from depression, lifted anxiety, or dealt with PTSD, now you're available to grow in other areas. For example, now may be the ideal time to start a highly nutritious diet and exercise program. Whatever it looks like for you, now's the time to go for it.

Finally, we recommend monitoring yourself, checking in with your moods and progress during the afterglow period and beyond. This will help you identify if and/or when you may want a *Maintenance* KAP session. Everyone differs, as some may want to revisit KAP within three to six months or once a year. There are two ways to monitor yourself:

- **Subjectively.** Sometimes you've got to trust your instincts. If you're feeling like it's time for another breakthrough, or to readjust your mindset, or you want to go deeper on an issue that may be clinging on, you may be ready to schedule a *Maintenance* session. Talking with your therapist can help you identify the next areas of healing, growth, or transformation desired.

MOOD TRACKER

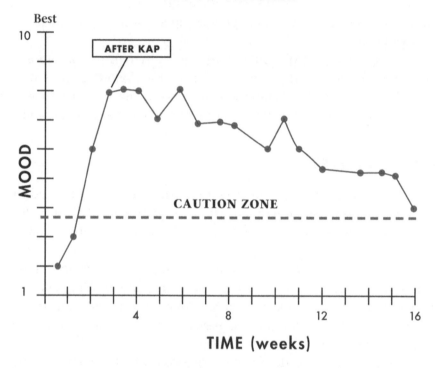

- **Objectively.** If subjective measures aren't enough to help you determine if/when another KAP session is warranted, we recommend tracking your mood over time to give you insight into any troubling trends that may arise. For a formal assessment of mood, you can reach out to your therapist and retake the two assessments we use to measure depression and anxiety, respectively: the PHQ-9 and the GAD-7. Your therapist can compare your current scores to your pretreatment scores. For an informal assessment, consider using a simple mood tracking chart that quantifies overall mood on a simple scale from 1 to 10—with 10 being the best. Make note of how you'd rate your overall mood on a scale of 1 to 10 before you began KAP, because approaching this number represents your caution zone. Make one in your journal, and plot your mood weekly. It's best to return fairly quickly for a *Maintenance* session after the mood begins dipping. Clients who wait more than six months for *Maintenance* are more likely to experience a return of depressive episodes. In some cases, that may also require a full regimen of six *Exploration* sessions as *Maintenance* versus a single *Exploration* session for a client who returns every four months.

SCHEDULE A *MAINTENANCE* SESSION

If or when you see your mood slipping into the "Caution Zone," or if you're seeking a breakthrough in a different area of your life, then you may want to consider scheduling a *Maintenance* session. A *Maintenance* session is simply an *Exploration* session that takes place after the initial course of treatment has been deemed successful. With the *Maintenance* protocol you can compress the *Preparation*, *Exploration*, and *Integration* sessions into a few days. Between you and your therapist, you decide how many *Exploration* and *Integration* sessions are necessary. Many times, people want to maintain their growth and healing by scheduling annual, biannual, or quarterly *Maintenance* sessions—much like a mental health checkup. Staying diligent on these checkups prevents the need for repeating multiple *Maintenance* sessions. For example, a person with severe depression will likely need only one *Maintenance* session if they do it quarterly. If they wait years and the depression has returned, they may need to start over and repeat the full cycle of six *Exploration* sessions. Additionally, you and your partner may decide to go through a couples session, or you may want to join a group. We also find that military veterans often want to experience KAP together. In the next few chapters, we've asked a few leading psychedelic therapists and experts to explain how these special populations benefit from the KAP experience.

PART III

KAP FOR SPECIAL POPULATIONS

CHAPTER 14

COUPLES: A TICKET TO DEEPER CONNECTION

Contributed by
Jeanine Souren, M.Sc., L.M.F.T., C.S.T.

As Ketamine-Assisted Psychotherapy (KAP) helps individuals find break-throughs in their lives, along with relieving stress, anxiety, and depression, we are finding benefits are amplified for couples seeking deeper connection. Couples experiencing KAP have the opportunity to address relational challenges, resolve past baggage, and prevent future pitfalls through slightly modified *Preparation*, *Exploration*, and *Integration* sessions. Not only do the individuals find the experience personally rewarding, but the protocols give each individual a chance to view their relationship in a whole new light. Clarity is gained. Communication is opened. Baggage is left behind.

While KAP doesn't magically wash all the couple's problems away, it does give both individuals insightful ways of looking at their problems—and at each other. Love and empathy are the most common feelings expressed after a session taking ketamine. Harnessing this openhearted feeling and focusing it through psychotherapy allows couples to climb a ladder to a higher level in their relationship.

Finding and maintaining a deep connection with your partner and nurturing a sense of belonging and mutual understanding sets the stage for what's ahead when doing KAP as a couple. The process will build trust, as couples become willing to let go and open to an enhanced level of intimacy. This can reshape the way the relationship is approached going forward.

By combining couples therapy with ketamine dosing, we can facilitate a safe and powerful way to reveal insight and honest conversations about relationship matters. Ketamine lowers defensive attitudes between partners, allowing underlying issues on both personal and relationship levels to be accessible. This enhanced vulnerability, openness, and honesty helps bridge the gap to deeper intimacy between partners.

More simply, clients share that they are able to see and be seen by their partner, to listen and to feel heard.

With KAP for couples, the basic protocol described in Part II of this book is augmented with therapeutic sessions designed to address the following:

- *Identity.* Discovering commonalities and differences in how each individual, and the couple, identify their relationship.

- *Unfinished business.* Identifying baggage from the past that may be weighing the relationship down.

- *Relationship dynamics.* How to let go of power and control to demonstrate selfless love and compassion in all situations.

- *Openness.* Being willing to increase knowledge of yourself and partner.

- *Relationship vision and values.* Gaining consensus for a mutual vision of hopes and desires for the future—along with an understanding of a new set of values to respect in the process.

- *Being present.* Ultimately being available, or present, in the relationship and attentive to each other's needs throughout life.

Another common issue that can be helped with KAP is related to sexual intimacy between the individuals. During therapy, couples may examine their views with their sexual relationship using the pleasure vs. purpose vs. fulfillment framework. The goal would be to find fulfillment. Sexual relationships that focus on achieving pleasure can become overly concerned with reaching orgasm or lead to infidelity. Comparatively, having sexual relations seeking a purpose, like to get pregnant or to prevent the spouse from going elsewhere, can diminish the ability to find sexual fulfillment. Sexual fulfillment is when physical pleasure occurs within the context of an intimate and loving relationship. By connecting with the couple's core values, intimacy can move from being pleasure- or purpose-oriented to an expression of love leading to fulfillment.

Using KAP for couples helps develop skills to restore trust, communicate and express feelings effectively, and understand and resolve differences. By undergoing the *Exploration* sessions, couples build deeper connections and understand why they get stuck in certain patterns—often as a result of past constructs, obstacles, and forces impacting the current behaviors in the relationship.

In the *Preparation* and *Integration* sessions, the partners work with a couples therapist to begin to understand the relationship dynamic, underlying hurts, and attachment styles. The objective is to improve communication skills and create a shared relationship vision, values, and desires for each other and the relationship.

During the *Preparation* sessions, the couples also decide with their therapist if they prefer to experience *Exploration* ketamine dosing sessions at the same time in separate rooms, or alternate the experience between them, one after the other. (See "Treatment Options" below.)

Using KAP for couples helps the individuals open up their minds to what's possible in the relationship, connect to what's important, and understand each other's perspectives with greater intimacy. The result is a fresh outlook on the relationship and the ability to navigate challenges moving forward.

WHAT CAN CLIENTS EXPECT FROM THE TREATMENT?

In short, clients can expect personal and relational growth.

Just like in individual KAP, couples will go through a medical screening and intake with the psychotherapist. This helps determine eligibility and which goals will be formulated prior to the *Preparation* session(s).

The number of sessions for *Preparation*, *Exploration*, and *Integration* is largely determined by the progress made in the relationship during the process. Typically, we recommend planning for six *Exploration* sessions, which last approximately one and a half to two hours each. Therefore, couples would have at least one *Preparation* session and six hours of *Integration* sessions, which are 50 to 60 minutes. While every couple and therapy differs, we tailor each session to each couple's unique dynamics. As with individual KAP, licensed medical professionals and a psychotherapist accompany the clients throughout the treatments. We also use self-reflection assignments prior to the *Exploration* sessions to assist the entire process. (See "What's the function of the assignments?")

When defenses have grown rock solid over the years, impasses and misunderstandings can lead to feelings of disconnect and resentment. Sometimes a major shift is necessary for relational growth, and couples KAP is uniquely suited to provide this. Many couples report that going through this unique experience together creates an even deeper bond.

WHO WOULD KAP FOR COUPLES BE APPROPRIATE FOR?

This program is quite intensive, so it's best for couples who are willing to do the deep work that is required of them. Most clients have had some prior experience with traditional psychotherapy and are ready to go even deeper. Since KAP creates and enhances a deep bond, it's not recommended for couples who have already decided to part ways or who need coparenting therapy. KAP for couples is an advanced approach to assist couples who are committed to their relationship and want to build a deeper connection. If the partners are open to diving deep into their own psyche and having honest conversations then significant breakthroughs can occur and help nurture the love and commitment in the relationship.

WHAT'S THE FUNCTION OF THE ASSIGNMENTS?

With the KAP for couples protocol, clients must do more than show up. There are self-reflection assignments designed to facilitate the therapeutic process. These are important parts of the protocol that enhance the synergy between the medicine and the therapy, maximizing the chance for the couple to attain a deeper connection and a stronger relationship. Self-reflection is the process of examining behavior or beliefs in a mindful way. Engaging in deliberate self-reflection helps the couple become aware of deeper mental and emotional issues that may be holding them back. Not only do they reveal personal insights, but also those as a couple, which prepares them for relational growth. Plus, these assignments will guide the couple and therapist to illuminate goals, intentions, and concerns, as well as expectations for the *Exploration* sessions. We also use the assignments to gather insights from the ketamine experience, which gives the therapist material to process during the *Integration* therapy sessions. Some assignments are completed as a couple to enhance openness and gain a deeper knowledge of each other's perspective. The assignments may include a discovery questionnaire, an openness exercise, identifying unfinished business, shared vision and values, listening and intimacy exercises, and a sexuality questionnaire.

Later in this chapter, there are five examples of self-reflection assignments we like to use for couples, including the following:

1. Start with the End in Mind

2. Drivers and Values

3. Intuitive Writing/Illustration Exercise

4. Unfinished Business

5. Sexuality Discovery

TREATMENT OPTIONS

There are three ways couples can experience the *Exploration* sessions. They may either (a) alternate turns taking the medicine in the same room, (b) have the ketamine experience at the same time but in adjacent rooms with different guides specializing in couples therapy, or (c) have the ketamine experience at the same time in the same room with one therapist. With the third option, the *Exploration* session tends to be longer, which needs to be accounted for.

When couples alternate turns, they are held, cradled, or supported by their partner. This offers a sense of safety and an "I've got you" feeling that may have been missing from childhood or the relationship. Holding your partner's hand is being granted entrance into the most vulnerable and sacred space of an individual—often where boundaries and ideals are exposed and protected fiercely.

Couples taking ketamine at the same time will each wake up from the experience and will meet in a comfortable lounge setting. Both are instructed how to navigate sharing their experience with each other. Couples often have clear access to the retrieved material and emotions during their inner journey just after the psychedelic experience ends—just like most people can remember their dreams in the first moments upon waking. Thus, journaling or drawing is encouraged. The next day, they'll have a couples *Integration* session with their therapist to review, analyze, and apply what was discovered. Or in the same room, they can use the ketamine as an empathogen and go directly into couples therapy upon "reentry."

The choice of what option is best for each unique relationship is based on personal preference and the therapist's advice during the *Preparation* session(s).

The couples intake questionnaire below is an example of how the therapist will help determine whether the ketamine dosing is done together in the same room, together in different rooms, or in alternate turns.

COUPLES INTAKE QUESTIONNAIRE: SAMPLE

A couples-focused questionnaire; fill out before intake interview with couples therapist:

1. Who in your partnership is the most concerned at this point about your relationship?

☐ I am

☐ My partner is

☐ Both

2. How concerned are you at this moment, on a scale of 0–10 (0 = not at all, 10 = very)?

3. Can you describe in a few lines why you believe this particular couples therapy approach could be helpful at this time?

4. Describe in about 10 lines what you are most concerned about.

5. On a scale of 0–10, when 0 means "not at all" concerned and 10 means "very much" concerned, how concerned do you think your partner is?

6. Can you describe in a few lines what you think your partner is worried about?

7. Can you describe in a few lines why you think your partner may or may not find this particular couples therapy approach helpful at this time?

8. Do you suffer from a mental health issue or diagnosis? If so, which one(s)?

9. Are you holding secrets that you don't want your partner to know?

10. Have you been in couples therapy before? If so, what worked and what didn't work?

11. How would you describe your self-regulation or ability to self-soothe?

12. How do you typically respond when you are in a conflict with your partner (withdraw, attack, surrender, minimize, stonewall, etc.)?

13. Do you try to control your partner? If so, how?

14. How do you disconnect from your partner?

15. How does your partner disconnect from you?

16. How do you try to avoid or get rid of painful feelings that are related to issues in the relationship?

17. Are you physically intimate with your partner? If so, how often?

18. Indicate the degree of happiness in your relationship (0–10, with 10 being the happiest) in terms of:

- Parenting
- Sex
- Parents-in-law
- Communication
- Household chores
- Meaningful time spent together

19. How would you describe the balance of power? Who is in charge? Who's in charge of what?

20. How would you describe your role in your relationship?

21. How were you different before this relationship?

22. Do you feel you can confide everything in your partner (0–10)?

23. Do you have a warm and comfortable relationship with your partner (0–10)?

24. Do you feel like a team with your partner (0–10)?

25. How are your (emotional) needs met by your partner (0–10)? Can you specify?

26. Do you believe your partner should change before you do? If so, what do you expect your partner to do?

27. How secure and stable do you feel in your relationship (0–10)?

28. Are you afraid your partner will leave you (yes/no)?

29. Do you worry about meeting your partner's expectations (yes/no)?

KAP FOR COUPLES: SELF-REFLECTION ASSIGNMENTS

Below are five examples of self-reflection assignments that may be used for couples.

1. Start with the end in mind.

- **Step A:** Visualize your life years from now, and answer the following: What would you like to have experienced, contributed, or achieved during your years on this planet? What would you like your legacy to be? How do you want to be remembered by your children? Think of either small or large achievements, either close to this moment or years down the road.

- **Step B:** Make a list of the things mentioned in step A and make an outline using the framework below, marking your progress next to each ambition.

#	Ambition: EXAMPLES	To do	Doing	Done
1	Happy relationship			
2	Write a book			
3	Traveled on each continent			

#	Ambition	To do	Doing	Done
1				
2				
3				
4				
5				
6				
7				
8				
9				
10				

2. Drivers and Values

- **Step A:** On separate sheets, each individual writes down what motivates them (drivers), what they care about, and what they think to be important (values). Each person identifies examples of decisions they made in the past and what drove those decisions.

- **Step B:** How would you prioritize these drivers and values (0 = low, 10 = high)?

Drivers/Domains	Value	Priority	Rank
Couples/intimate relationships	to be a loving partner	10	6
Parenting			
Family relations			
Social relations			
Employment			
Education and training			
Recreation			
Spirituality			
Citizenship/community			
Health/physical well-being			

- Rank each driver/domain based on the importance you place on working on them right now, with 1 being the most timely.

- Share your sheets and compare. Consider where you have shared dreams; talk about your vision and your shared vision.

- Then, create a shared-values list for your relationship: Which drivers and values resonate with the relationship? See if you can find three to six shared drivers and values.

3. Intuitive Writing/Illustration Exercise

What sort of partner would you like to be in an intimate relationship? What personal qualities would you like to develop? What sort of relationship would you like to build? How would you interact with your partner if you were the "ideal you" in this relationship?

Alternatively, make a drawing(s) of your relationship and vision of:

- The past
- The present
- The future

4. Unfinished Business

Your early experiences shape what you believe about the world and your place in it. In this exercise, couples examine any attachments from the past that are causing problems in the present.

- Identify the DRAIN in Your Relationship[1]

    D: Disconnection, R: Reactivity, A: Avoidance, I: Inside your mind, N: Neglecting values

    Disconnection: How do I disconnect from my partner? (E.g., Do I get bored, irritable, or stop listening? Do I go cold and distant? Do I close off/shut down? Am I distracted rather than present?)
    How does my partner disconnect from me?

    Reactivity: How do I react impulsively or automatically, without stopping to consider what I am doing? (E.g., Do I yell, snap, swear, storm off, say hurtful things, criticize, blame, accuse, sneer, jeer?)
    How does my partner react impulsively or automatically?

    Avoidance: How do I try to avoid or get rid of my painful feelings that are related to the issues in this relationship? (E.g., Do I use drugs, alcohol, food, cigarettes? Do I withdraw or stay away from my partner? Do I try to distract myself with TV, computers, books, or going out? Do I avoid talking to my partner about the issue?)
    How does my partner seem to avoid or get rid of painful feelings?

Inside your mind: How do I get trapped inside my mind? (E.g., Do I worry about the future, dwell on the past, relive old hurts, rehash old arguments, stew over everything that's wrong with my partner? Do I get caught up in judgment, blame, criticism? Do I get caught up in thoughts of rejection, betrayal, abandonment, or being controlled?)

How does my partner seem to get trapped inside his/her mind?

Neglecting values: What core values do I neglect, forget about, or act inconsistently with when I am disconnected, reactive, avoidant, or inside my mind? (E.g., Do I lose touch with values such as being loving, kind, caring, generous, compassionate, supportive, fun-loving, easygoing, sensual, affectionate?)

What core values does my partner seem to neglect, forget about, or act inconsistently with?

5. Sexuality Discovery

Use these questions for a better understanding of your sex life. Take time to answer each question on your own (both partners will do this individually).

You can keep these answers to yourself or share them with your partner when you are ready.

Questions

1. How has my sex life developed over time and in my relationship?

2. What does sex mean to me?

3. How do I communicate what I like and don't like?

4. How does my upbringing play a role in me as a sexual being?

5. What is my sexual strength and weakness?

6. How do we "talk" in bed without words? Who starts? Who stops?

7. How do we end our lovemaking?

8. How comfortable am I with my body?

9. How can I prioritize sex in our relationship? What's in the way?

10. What is the connection between sex and power in our relationship?

11. If I could write a song about our sex life, what type of music would I choose?

12. Do I share sexual fantasies with my partner?

13. What have I never tried (sexually) in our relationship that I would like to discover?

14. How often do I have solo sex in a week, and what do I aim for? (E.g., Pleasure, peak, or something else?)

15. Finish the sentence: Sex and love . . .

16. If I were to describe my orgasm with a metaphor (E.g., a butterfly, thunder, lightning), I would say . . .

Creative Assignment: Using colored pencils, markers, or crayons, draw your current sex life and your desired future one.

Couples considering the KAP protocol can be assured that there is an exciting adventure ahead—one with both personal and relational insights that can be life-changing. By integrating ketamine medicine with advanced therapeutic techniques, massive insights can be gained in a relatively short time. This is not a marital workshop weekend with short-lived experiences. Rather, KAP for couples has the potential to significantly improve the relationship forever.

The dynamic created with KAP for couples can be created in group settings as well, where insights from others can be shared for mutual benefit. Next, we have outlined how to extend the KAP protocol to support various group therapy settings, and have seen incredible results.

Jeanine Souren brings more than 15 years' experience as a registered and accredited professional psychologist and sexologist. Specializing in relationships, family systems, and helping couples find a deeper connection, she uses a variety of techniques including Psychedelic-Assisted Psychotherapy. Based in Amsterdam, Jeanine works with clients from around the world. Connect with Jeanine at jeaninesouren.com.

CHAPTER 15

GROUPS: THE MULTIPLIER EFFECT

Contributed by
Sabina Pillai, M.A., and Robin Banister

While ketamine offers a highly personalized awakening, something amazing—the multiplier effect—can occur when the protocol is done in a group setting. Numerous studies, as well as our own clinical work leading ketamine groups, show groups provide an opportunity for individuals to learn from each other, form unique bonds, reduce fears, and ultimately extend the therapeutic benefits.

It's probably no real surprise, since the use of psychedelic and plant medicines in group settings has a long history, owing to Indigenous cultural and spiritual traditions found in South and Central America, Africa, Asia, and Europe.[1]

Group therapy in Western contexts developed in the early 1940s and has evolved and adapted to meet the needs of a variety of clients in many different settings. Irvin D. Yalom, a psychotherapist and longtime advocate for group psychotherapy, found that groups can facilitate healing and growth through instillation of hope, appreciating the universality of human experience, interpersonal learning and socialization, psychoeducation, altruism and reciprocity, and corrective emotional and relational experiences.[2]

Given the prolific levels of isolation and disconnection being experienced today, where anxiety and depression is often coupled with a loss of meaning and purpose in people's lives, ketamine holds incredible promise for healing in group psychotherapy settings. Similarly to classic psychedelics, ketamine's unique properties can offer a way to transform old ways of thinking and operating in our lives. Recent research suggests that group use of ketamine allows individuals to be more open and vulnerable with others, creating the possibility for healing attachment wounds and practicing new, healthier ways of connecting with others.[3] Individuals in group therapy witness and learn from others' healing journeys, consider many different perspectives and life experiences, and share unconditional positive regard. Through the group, members may start to see how one's personal transformation and collective liberation are deeply intertwined. Bridging Western science and Indigenous spiritual traditions through group psychedelic-assisted psychotherapy can offer a hybrid approach that may resonate with an array of individuals and connect them with what they feel may be missing in their lives.

Experiencing ketamine-assisted therapy together as a group can enhance the positive effects when conducted in a clinical setting, especially for those struggling with anxiety, depression, and trauma. Having a skilled team of licensed professionals administering ketamine in a comfortable and safe setting while one's vitals are monitored can further facilitate one's ability to trust and let go into the group experience. Similar to individual psychedelic psychotherapy, you may experience heightened emotions, less defensiveness, and increased feelings of vulnerability. And yet, allowing ourselves to risk being vulnerable in a thoughtfully curated, supportive community can be exactly what's necessary to repair wounds stemming from past relationships and offer the opportunity to build fellowship among like-minded individuals on similar journeys of healing and transformation.

TYPES OF GROUPS

While there can be benefits to group experiences with members from different sociocultural, economic, age, gender, and sexuality backgrounds in terms of cultivating openness and appreciating commonalities in the human experience, group therapy can be especially potent when curated for specific subgroups. One essential ingredient of the group experience is the cultivation of trust and safety in a relatively short period of time. For longer, process-oriented groups, these elements will have time to grow and build; however, when considering current uses of psychedelics in group settings (e.g., clinics, retreats, ceremonies), common factors among group members can rapidly accelerate feelings of trust, safety, intimacy, and connection.

Groups composed of individuals with similar life experiences could especially benefit from collective healing experiences. For example, groups catering to BIPOC, LGBTQ, veterans, sexual assault survivors, grief, substance use, men's and women's issues, and individuals with specific mental health conditions can offer incredible opportunities to healing among others who have faced similar challenges in life.

PROTOCOL DIFFERENCES

During the *Preparation* session, the group will meet together with the group therapist. To help the participants prepare to engage in a group therapy experience, it is vital to establish a clear understanding of the expectations and boundaries. This helps create an environment of safety and trust, two ingredients that are essential for people to be able to enter into this process with an open mindset. During this phase of treatment, the structure of the sessions is outlined and expectations are communicated. This includes informed consent, regular attendance and punctuality, full presence in integration sessions, confidentiality, and a code of ethics that we ask everyone to abide by during the treatment process. Every individual needs to agree on these parameters in order to foster a safe experience. All group members have an opportunity to introduce themselves and share their experiences, values, concerns, and intentions for treatment. Members will typically find that there are some commonalities among them, whether that be in their current struggles or hopes for the future. This begins the process of creating community, which can be another powerful medicine in and of itself. We want to emphasize this point. In many cases, the power of community that people find through group experiences has greater lasting impact and effect than the ketamine sessions.

On the day of the ketamine experience (*Exploration* session), clients arrive at the clinic and get checked in by the medical team. The clients and therapist convene in a common space as a group. Group members share how they are feeling as well as their intention for the day. Clients are offered a meditation to allow them to settle into the present and connect with their bodies prior to their journey. Once this connection has been made, the clients are given a weighted blanket and encouraged to settle into their recliner or daybed. The dosing session begins by listening to a thoughtfully curated selection of music meant to facilitate relaxation and presence. Members are administered ketamine either via an intramuscular (IM) injection or a sublingual lozenge. They are also encouraged to wear eyeshades and headphones for the duration of their journey. The session takes around two hours, but some flexibility is given to those who may need some extra time. Once everyone has completed their journey, they are offered refreshments and encouraged to take some time to personally reflect on their journey by journaling or drawing.

Afterward, all group members and the therapist sit together in a circle and are encouraged to share as much as they are comfortable about their experience. Typically, the residual effects of the ketamine help soften our defenses, and folks are more willing to be vulnerable with one another. Many times, members share their insights or frustrations, elements of their journey, their personal history, or how they were impacted by others in the room. Members tend to feel deeply validated by hearing their stories echoed in others and begin to truly understand that they are not alone. In this process of sharing, the individual is being witnessed and accepted in what they may have thought, up until that moment, was unacceptable.

In Yalom's perspective, this confirmation of a client's feelings is a powerful source of relief, and can result in them feeling more allied with the world.[4] Clients have voiced in group sessions, "I had no idea other people had similar narratives running through their minds. I thought I was the only person in the world who had these thoughts." Reflecting and sharing is a deeply important part of the *Integration* session, as it allows the experience to become more concrete while providing a greater opportunity to connect with and learn from the other members. The therapist encourages discussion among the group, and ensures that there is a relatively even exchange among participants and that boundaries are being respected. The session then concludes with an exercise to acknowledge the conclusion of the circle.

Another valuable aspect of experiencing ketamine as a group in a clinical setting is the presence of a qualified, licensed group therapist who facilitates the entire experience. Facilitators should have training and experience in facilitating groups, they should be present and aware, and they should be skilled at holding space with both warmth and groundedness. Ideally, group therapists will strive to balance both structure and flexibility. Structure is essential to build trust, safety, and connection among group members prior to their journey as well as during integration support and processing following the journey. Flexibility is important in order to organically support the unfolding process emerging among group members during the treatment and respond to any challenges that may arise during that process within or between individuals in the group.

We believe the optimal environment for groups doing ketamine therapy is the same as for individuals—a safe, cozy space with comfortable seating, music, tissues, and low lighting during the treatment. Additionally, things like blankets, daybeds, incense, and refreshments during post-journey reflection can serve to enhance the experience. The facility should approach the creation of the group with thoughtfulness to ensure cohesiveness among members and that those not suited for the group environment are screened.

Ketamine groups may also provide a slightly lower cost for individuals, although the extent of each individual's therapy may affect the overall fees. In the end, ketamine delivers a powerful opportunity to create new possibilities for personal growth. And when individuals combine the experience with others in a group, the results can be multiplied.

Sabina Pillai, M.A., is a registered psychotherapist trained in clinical and counseling psychology and Buddhist psychology at the University of Toronto. She has worked in mental health for more than a decade in individual and group psychotherapy, conducting research on non-ordinary states of consciousness and psychedelics, and published peer reviewed articles on addictions and mindfulness. She currently works as the senior lead psychotherapist at Field Trip, offering ketamine and psychedelic-assisted psychotherapy.

Robin Banister is a registered psychotherapist specializing in existential integrative psychotherapy, helping clients navigate the oftentimes transpersonal nature of their psychedelic-assisted therapy experiences. Her background in psilocybin research adds to her knowledge of preparation and integration work that is essential to the healing process. She is currently working as a ketamine-assisted psychotherapist at Field Trip. Based in Toronto, Robin works with clients from Ontario, Canada, and beyond. Connect with Robin at robinbanistertherapy.com.

CHAPTER 16

VETERANS: HEALING WITH COMMON BONDS

In 2010, I was blown up in Afghanistan. We had been setting up a military observation post, and on the way back we were struck by an IED (improvised explosive device). I had shrapnel wounds to my stomach, right lower leg, hand, and another piece went in my ear and through the back of my head. My fire team partner sustained life-threatening injuries that resulted in his death eight days later.

I was able to recover from the physical wounds, although a piece of shrapnel still sits next to my spine. But the mental toll is another story. I suffered from night terrors that led to insomnia, anxiety, depression, and always being hypervigilant. I hoped that with time it would go away, but it didn't. It was debilitating.

I decided to try Ketamine-Assisted Psychotherapy after hearing from other vets who said it helped them manage pain and concentration, along with their anxiety. I'd never taken any kind of psychedelic before so I was pretty nervous. During my first [ketamine] session, a floodgate of emotions opened up, which had been building for quite some time. I was transported back to Afghanistan where we got blown up, rifle in hand. I was walking through the old stomping grounds and ran into my fire team partner who died from the blast. He told me he'd been with me the whole time. I also saw several other comrades who had committed suicide post-tour. I engaged in conversations with them, which provided me with a sense of tranquility.

Through my experience with ketamine therapy, I was finally able to address the hard stuff, and unpack it in a real and meaningful way. Nothing has helped me with PTSD as much as this. My general anxiety and depression have subsided, and I'm much happier. Participating in Ketamine-Assisted Psychotherapy was the best decision I've made in my recovery journey.

These days I'm feeling positive and optimistic. I used to indulge in substances to help numb my pain, and that's something I haven't felt the need to do since my ketamine therapies. I've since moved to Toronto and have a new routine that includes yoga, swimming, and going to the gym. I finally feel like I can stand on my own with gratitude, and I remind myself daily that I haven't come this far only to come this far.

—Grant, actual patient from Field Trip

The term *warrior* can bring connotations of being brave, tough, lethal, and never admitting to weakness. Serving in the military protecting their country is a proud honor. However, all too often veterans of war come home stuck in a warrior-robot mode, bringing with them haunting memories of gruesome experiences in the battlefield, and unable to flip the switch of performing from a warrior mindset into docile civilian life. The warrior has a new war, an internal battle with fears of letting down their guard and being seen as cowardly, vulnerable, and weak.

Adam Wright, a former U.S. Navy SEAL and clinic operations manager at Field Trip in Washington, D.C., explains that SEALs are taught to remain in a hyper-vigilant state, and to disassociate from their mind, body, and emotions. There's no room for empathy because the military is designed to harm human life. "As a SEAL, your central purpose is built around killing other people. That's the world you live in, and it comes with a cost. War zones are gray moral zones. You have to live with the fact that the job requires that warriors murder, which is essentially a criminal activity in the civilian world."

No wonder veterans of war come home different. The human brain is sensitive to stimuli while creating memories that cannot be erased. Becoming a warrior is like trying to remove a person's humanness. Due to their experiences, whether or not they were in combat, veterans bring post-traumatic stress disorder (PTSD), traumatic brain injuries (TBI), depression, and anxiety to the home front. They struggle with compartmentalizing their trauma outside of their lives in uniform. After identifying as a warrior, it's nearly impossible to retrain the brain that you're anything else. And war veterans aren't the only ones suffering with this identity crisis—often frontline workers and professional athletes also think of themselves as warriors with battles they engage in daily.

With ketamine, warriors find immediate relief from these identities while being provided an opportunity to see their experiences and memories from a new perspective. Adam compares the protocol to returning to "base camp," where veterans can come off the mountaintops of war and find a place to recover, regroup, and regain perspective. The term *base camp* has become the code word for the protocol offered to veterans and other "warriors" through Field Trip.

Warriors can go through the Base Camp protocol individually, or in a group setting where the overall cost for the ketamine therapy decreases. In Canada, Veterans Affairs Canada covers virtually all of the costs for this treatment.

Adam said the group protocol helps warriors reintegrate into society because they can temporarily lower their guards and experiment with being vulnerable in front of others, perhaps for the first time.

"Veterans don't trust other people enough and often feel like they have to wear a mask in their community. It's a unique challenge because warriors are taught to put on a persona around their teammates," he said. "With this, they can learn to take off their body armor, put down their gun, and find their true selves."

By using the ketamine protocol together, their common bonds pave the way to healing individually.

Brian Fernandes, a registered social worker with the Ontario College of Social Workers specializing in psychedelic-assisted psychotherapy, has worked with more than 44 military veterans who have gone through the ketamine therapy protocol through Field Trip in Toronto. He said that literally 100 percent of those he has worked with report having been diagnosed with PTSD, depression, anxiety, or addiction. And these conditions don't come in a silo. Each brings challenges with relationships, sleep, or conflicts with the law.

Brian, also an infantry officer in the Canadian Army Reserve, offers highly relevant experience helping men and women become warriors and develop resilience. Veterans have been taught to live by a code, or mantra, that the mission comes first, followed by your team, then yourself. From the beginning of the intake procedures, Brian says veterans living in the civilian world need to be able to reverse this thinking so they put themselves and their mental health first, then they are better able to be of service to their family, friends, and colleagues and whatever "mission" they embark on.

The Base Camp protocol doesn't differ too much from what we've discussed for groups in the previous chapter, with the same *Preparation, Exploration,* and *Integration* sessions. However, we've seen some veterans who prefer to have their *Preparation* sessions individually, rather than in a group. Brian says this helps build trust and camaraderie between the veteran and clinician—which in Field Trip's case is typically another veteran like Brian. This also helps the veteran ease into the experience, learning to be vulnerable with their true thoughts and feelings with another person. Becoming open and willing to gain insight from ketamine means the veteran may have to let down their guard, which isn't always easy but is always beneficial.

For example, during a ketamine session with a veteran group, Brian said one of the members began drooling while the medication was being administered, so much so that it soaked his shirt and caused him to feel cold, preventing the ketamine from producing its intended effects. He felt embarrassed and angry, like he had been shortchanged by the experience, and threatened to leave the clinic immediately.

"I know you expected to achieve healing but that was interrupted. It wasn't anybody's fault, but it still interrupted the experience," Brian told him. "Let me suggest taking a moment to sit with these feelings, and bring it to the group for discussion."

He did, and something amazing happened.

Instead of facing his disappointment alone, he found acceptance and support from comrades who were able to empathize and identify with his emotional experience, their own journeys being paved with numerous frustrations and barriers. This paved the way for disclosing feelings of guilt and shame, which was also common among each of the veterans in the group. The power of honesty to share in a safe space with like-minded brothers-in-arms led to a powerful experience after all.

Traumatic memories can't be erased. Turning off the warrior-robot mindset is not easy. Learning a new mantra to put yourself first may seem counterintuitive to a veteran. But warriors are human. With ketamine, and through common bonds and camaraderie, we can help lift the weight of the war and open a window for healing to come in. Then a whole new world opens, which can mean a future filled with awe and wonder.

EPILOGUE

From Final Stop to Send-Off

All journeys have a destination. By the time you're reading this, your flight will have landed and you'll have arrived at your destination, at least for this leg of this journey. You've done the work. You've transformed. Your metamorphosis is underway.

Just as the excitement of getting off an airplane breeds anticipation, we expect you'll find yourself eager to enjoy the possibilities now opened to you.

From us to you, please now take a moment, a day, a week, a month to stop and take it in. Appreciate everything that's happened, and is happening, within and around you. In this day and age, we rarely give ourselves permission to breathe, let alone appreciate, celebrate, and honor our successes and our victories. So breathe. Appreciate. Celebrate. It matters.

If you need more inspiration, here are some of the things you may wish to celebrate:

- You now have some of the most in-depth knowledge and understanding about ketamine and ketamine-assisted therapy of just about anyone, save for the most knowledgeable experts in the field.

- You will have tools and skills that can equip you to handle and respond to just about anything that life will throw your way.

- The tightness in your chest, that anxiety that you never really knew you were carrying around, feels lighter or has disappeared entirely. You may even find moments of warmth and ease in your chest that you probably hadn't experienced since childhood.

- Smiles and laughter come more easily—as do tears of joy and sorrow. Our highs feel higher and our lows may feel lower as we start to loosen the grip on the emotions and beliefs we've held so tightly for so long.

- Energy levels increase as we dedicate less time and effort to trying to just hold on, and lean into flow states and acceptance.

- Those things that have triggered you in the past may not trigger you anymore. Or maybe they do but it's not quite as severe. Or maybe you're just now able to notice and be aware of the trigger and the narrative that causes it. With that knowledge you feel empowered. That thing that once seemed like a life sentence of hurt or anger or sadness or anxiety now seems like just a hurdle.

If you're looking for the word to sum up the feelings around these achievements, we'd suggest *wonderful*, in the truest essence of its meaning—full of wonder. And there is more that lies ahead.

Though we've arrived at your destination, your journey is not over. The work you've done throughout this book has opened new possibilities.

Your journey will continue. Life is motion. Life is growth. More moments of joy and fulfillment are now within grasp. And when you're in those moments, when you're feeling empowered and motivated to continue on your journey, lean into it. Delve deeper, explore yourself further.

Sometimes your journey is going to be full of what we will kindly call "unexpected growth opportunities." As has happened to both of us, there will be occasions when you turn the page on a chapter of your life or journey and you'll reach the end of that book. And there will be times when turning the page opens up not only a new chapter but an entirely new book. New challenges will arise. This can be daunting or frustrating. It certainly happens to us, and it is absolutely okay. When these moments happen, have compassion for yourself. Give yourself a break.

Every time that voice in your head tells you all of the things that you "should" do, remind yourself that it's okay to not be okay or motivated at times. Remind yourself of the graph below. When you're riding the highs of the roller coaster, full of energy, go all in. When it gets bumpy, take a pause.

We are on the exact same journey as you. We go through those ups and downs just as you do. We feel daunted sometimes, just as you will. But we are here to support you. In fact, there is a whole growing world of people embracing the power of ketamine and psychedelic-assisted therapies ready to support you. You are now not only finding greater connection to yourself, you've joined a global community breaking through with these therapies who are eager to support you as well. That's the remarkable thing about these experiences: When you feel more connected to yourself, you become more connected to the entire world around you, and you'll quickly find people in your community who are discovering the same thing and cheering for you, just as you start cheering for them.

We opened this book with a bold claim that we are not only on the brink of revolutionizing mental health but are also opening people up to a new world of possibilities. After reading through this book, and doing the work, we hope you now know why we are confidently proclaiming this to be true, and why we are dedicating our lives to helping these powerful therapies reach more people. Life has never been so full of opportunity, especially after you've sorted through the ketamine experience. We encourage you to continue and grab on to what's ahead.

ENDNOTES

INTRODUCTION

1. Goodwin, G. M., et al. "Emotional blunting with antidepressant treatments: A survey among depressed patients." *Journal of Affective Disorders* 221 (2017): 31–35. https://doi.org/10.1016/j.jad.2017.05.048.

2. Price, J., Cole, V., and Goodwin, G. M. "Emotional side-effects of selective serotonin reuptake inhibitors: qualitative study." *British Journal of Psychiatry* 195, no. 3 (2009): 211–7. https://doi.org/10.1192/bjp.bp.108.051110. Aydemir, E. O., Asian, E., and Yazici, M. K. "SSRI induced apathy syndrome." *Psychiatry and Behavioral Sciences* 8, no. 2 (2018): 63–70.https://doi.org/10.5455/PBS.20180115111230.

CHAPTER 1

1. World Health Organization. WHO Model List of Essential Medicines, 2019. https://apps.who.int/iris/bitstream/handle/10665/325771/WHO-MVP-EMP-IAU-2019.06-eng.pdf.

2. Berman, R. M., et al. "Antidepressant effects of ketamine in depressed patients." *Biological Psychiatry* 47, no. 4 (2000): 351–354. https://doi.org/10.1016/S0006-3223(99)00230-9.

3. Henderson, T. A. "Practical application of the neuroregenerative properties of ketamine: real world treatment experience." *Neural Regeneration Research* 11, no. 2 (2016): 195–200. https://doi.org/10.4103/1673-5374.177708.

4. Palhano-Fontes, F., et al. "The psychedelic state induced by Ayahuasca modulates the activity and connectivity of the Default Mode Network." Edited by Dewen Hu. *PLoS One* 10, no. 2 (February 2015). https://doi.org/10.1371/journal.pone.0118143.

5. Carhart-Harris, R., et al. "The entropic brain: A theory of conscious states informed by neuroimaging research with psychedelic drugs." *Frontiers in Human Neuroscience* (2014). https://doi.org/10.3389/fnhum.2014.00020.

CHAPTER 2

1. Bahji, A., Vazquez, G. H., and Zarate Jr., C. A. "Comparative efficacy of racemic ketamine and esketamine for depression: a systematic review and meta-analysis." *Journal of Affective Disorders* 278 (2021): 542–555. https://doi.org/10.1016/j.jad.2020.09.071.

2. Robson, M., et al. "Evaluation of sigma (σ) receptors in the antidepressant-like effects of ketamine in vitro and in vivo." *European Neuropsychopharmacology* 22, no. 4 (2012): 308–317.

3. Yang, C., et al. "R-ketamine: a rapid-onset and sustained antidepressant without psychotomimetic side effects." *Translational Psychiatry* 5, no. 9 (2015): 1–11. https://doi .org/10.1038/tp.2015.136.

4. Muraresku, Brian C. *The Immortality Key: The Secret History of the Religion with No Name.* (New York: St. Martin's Press, 2020).

5. Bleckwenn, W. J. "Narcosis as therapy in neuropsychiatric conditions." *JAMA* 95, no. 16 (1930): 1168–1171. https://doi.org/10.1001/jama.1930.02720160028009.

6. Berman, R. M., et al. "Antidepressant effects of ketamine in depressed patients." *Biological Psychiatry* 47, no. 4 (February 15, 2000): 351–54. https://doi.org/10.1016 /s0006-3223(99)00230-9.

7. Khorramzadeh, E., and Lofty, A. O. "The use of ketamine in psychiatry." *Psychosomatics* 14, no. 6 (November–December 1973): 344–46. https://doi.org/10.1016/S0033 -3182(73)71306-2.

8. Krystal, J. H., Karper, L. P., Seibyl, J. P., Freeman, G. K., Delaney, R., Bremner, J. D., & Charney, D. S. (1994). "Subanesthetic effects of the noncompetitive NMDA antagonist, ketamine, in humans." *Archives of General Psychiatry* 51, no. 3 (March 1994): 199–214. https://doi.org/10.1001/archpsyc.1994.03950030035004.

9. Berman, R. M., Cappiello, A., Anand, A., Oren, D. A., Heninger, G. R., Charney, D. S., & Krystal, J. H. (2000). "Antidepressant effects of ketamine in depressed patients." *Biological Psychiatry*, 47(4), 351-354. https://doi.org/10.1016/s0006-3223(99)00230-9.

10. Moda-Sava, R. N., et al. "Sustained rescue of prefrontal circuit dysfunction by antidepressant-induced spine formation." *Science* 364, no. 6436. https://doi.org/10.1126 /science.aat8078.

11. Roquet, S., et al. *The Existential Through Psychodysleptics—A New Psychotherapy.* (Mexico City: Asociacion Albert Schweitzer, 1971).

12. Fontana, A. "Terapia antidepresiva con Ci 581 (ketamine)." *Acta Psiquiatrica y Psicologica de America Latina* 4 (1974): 20–32.

13. Khorramzadeh, E., and Lofty, A. O. *Psychosomatics* 14, 344–46.

14. Krupitsky, E. M., et al. "The combination of psychedelic and aversive approaches in alcoholism treatment: the affective contra-attribution method." *Alcoholism Treatment Quarterly* 9, no. 1 (1992): 99–105.

15. Krupitsky, E. M., and Grinenko, A. Y. "Ketamine psychedelic therapy (KPT): a review

of the results of ten years of research." *Journal of Psychoactive Drugs* 29, no. 2 (1997): 165–183. https://doi.org/10.1080/02791072.1997.10400185.

16. Kolp, Eli, et al. "Ketamine psychedelic psychotherapy: Focus on its pharmacology, phenomenology, and clinical applications." *International Journal of Transpersonal Studies* 33, no. 2 (2014): 84–140. https://doi.org/10.24972/ijts.2014.33.2.84.

CHAPTER 3

1. Salomon, R. M., et al. "Lack of behavioral effects of monoamine depletion in healthy subjects." *Biological Psychiatry* 41, no. 1 (January 1, 1997): 58–64. https://doi .org/10.1016/0006-3223(95)00670-2.

2. Rush, A. J., et al. "Comparative efficacy of cognitive therapy and pharmacotherapy in the treatment of depressed outpatients." *Cognitive Therapy and Research* 1 (1977): 17–37. https://doi.org/10.1007/BF01173502.

3. Hillhouse, T. M., and Porter, J. H. "A brief history of the development of antidepressant drugs: from monoamines to glutamate." *Experimental and Clinical Psychopharmacology* 23, no. 1 (February 2015): 1–21. https://doi.org/10.1037/a0038550.

4. Krupitsky, E. M., et al. "Metabolism of biogenic amines induced by alcoholism narcopsychotherapy with ketamine administration." *Biogenic Amines* 7, no. 6 (1990): 577–582.

5. du Jardin, K. G., et al. "Potential involvement of serotonergic signaling in ketamine's antidepressant actions: A critical review." *Progress in Neuro-Psychopharmacology & Biological Psychiatry* 71 (November 2016): 27–38. https://doi.org/10.1016/j. pnpbp.2016.05.007.

6. Garay, R. P., et al. "Investigational drugs in recent clinical trials for treatment-resistant depression." *Expert Review of Neurotherapeutics* 17, no. 6 (June 2017): 593–609. https:// doi.org/10.1080/14737175.2017.1283217.

7. Moda-Sava, R. N., et al. "Sustained rescue of prefrontal circuit dysfunction by antidepressant-induced spine formation." *Science* 364, no. 6436. https://doi.org/10.1126 /science.aat8078.

8. Karege, F., et al. "Decreased serum brain-derived neurotrophic factor levels in major depressed patients." *Psychiatry Research* 109, no. 2 (March 2002): 143–48. https://doi .org/10.1016/s0165-1781(02)00005-7.

9. Garcia, L. S. B., et al. "Acute administration of ketamine induces antidepressant-like effects in the forced swimming test and increases BDNF levels in the rat hippocampus." *Progress in Neuro-Psychopharmacology & Biological Psychiatry* 32, no. 1 (January 2008): 140–44. https://doi.org/10.1016/j.pnpbp.2007.07.027.

10. Haile, C. N., et al. "Plasma brain derived neurotrophic factor (BDNF) and response to ketamine in treatment-resistant depression." *International Journal of Neuropsychopharmacology* 17, no. 2 (February 2014): 331–36. https://doi.org/10.1017 /S1461145713001119.

11. Raichle, M. E., et al. "A default mode of brain function." *Proceedings of the National Academy of Sciences* 98, no. 2 (2001): 676–82. https://doi.org/10.1073/pnas.98.2.676.

12. Spreng, R. N. "The fallacy of a 'task-negative' network." *Frontiers in Psychology* 3 (2012): 145. https://doi.org/10.3389/fpsyg.2012.00145.

13. Spreng, R. N., et al. "The default network of the human brain is associated with perceived social isolation." *Nature Communications* 11, no. 1 (2020): 6393. https://doi .org/10.1038/s41467-020-20039-w.

14. Zhou, H. X., et al. "Rumination and the default mode network: Meta-analysis of brain imaging studies and implications for depression." *NeuroImage* 206 (February 2020): 116287. https://doi.org/10.1016/j.neuroimage.2019.116287.

15. Creswell, J. D., et al. "Alterations in resting-state functional connectivity link mindfulness meditation with reduced interleukin-6: a randomized controlled trial." *Biological Psychiatry* 80, no. 1 (2016): 53–61. https://doi.org/10.1016/j.biopsych.2016.01.008. Huang, W., et al. "Characterizing acupuncture stimuli using brain imaging with FMRI-a systematic review and meta-analysis of the literature." *PloS One* 7, no. 4 (April 2012): e32960. https://doi.org/10.1371/journal.pone.0032960.

16. Scheidegger, M., et al. "Ketamine decreases resting state functional network connectivity in healthy subjects: implications for antidepressant drug action." *PloS One* 7, no. 9 (September 2012): e44799. https://doi.org/10.1371/journal.pone.0044799.

17. Lebedev, A. V., et al. "Finding the self by losing the self: Neural correlates of ego-dissolution under psilocybin." *Human Brain Mapping* 36, no. 8 (May 2015): 3137–53. https://doi.org/10.1002/hbm.22833.

18. Lynall, M. E., et al. "Peripheral blood cell–stratified subgroups of inflamed depression." *Biological psychiatry* 88, no. 2 (2020): 185–96. https://doi.org/10.1016 /j.biopsych.2019.11.017.

19. Pedraz-Petrozzi, B., Neumann, E., and Sammer, G. "Pro-inflammatory markers and fatigue in patients with depression: A case-control study." *Scientific Reports* 10, no. 1 (2020): 1–12. https://doi.org/10.1038/s41598-020-66532-6.

20. Bhutta, A. T., et al. "Ketamine as a neuroprotective and anti-inflammatory agent in children undergoing surgery on cardiopulmonary bypass: a pilot randomized, double-blind, placebo-controlled trial." *Pediatric Critical Care Medicine* 13, no. 3 (May 2012): 328–37. https://doi.org/10.1097/PCC.0b013e31822f18f9.

21. Wu, G. J., et al. "Ketamine inhibits tumor necrosis factor-α and interleukin-6 gene expressions in lipopolysaccharide-stimulated macrophages through suppression of toll-like receptor 4-mediated c-Jun N-terminal kinase phosphorylation and activator protein-1 activation." *Toxicology and Applied Pharmacology* 228, no. 1 (April 2008): 105–13. https://doi.org/10.1016/j.taap.2007.11.027. Al Jurdi, R. K., Swann, A., and Mathew, S. J. "Psychopharmacological agents and suicide risk reduction: ketamine and other approaches." *Current Psychiatry Reports* 17, no. 10 (October 2015): 1–10. https://doi.org/10.1007/s11920-015-0614-9.

22. Ibid.

CHAPTER 4

1. MAPS Public Benefit Corp. "MAPS' Phase 3 Trial of MDMA-Assisted Therapy for PTSD Achieves Highly Statistically Significant Results for Patients with Severe, Chronic PTSD," news, press release, May 3, 2021, https://mapspublicbenefit.com/press-releases/maps-phase-3-trial.

2. Isaacson, W. *Steve Jobs* (New York: Simon & Schuster, 2021), Chapter 3.

3. Robbins, T. *Wild Ducks Flying Backward* (New York: Bantam Books, 2005).

CHAPTER 5

1. Al Jurdi, R. K., Swann, A., and Mathew, S. J. "Psychopharmacological agents and suicide risk reduction: ketamine and other approaches." *Current Psychiatry Reports* 17, no. 10 (October 2015): 1–10. https://doi.org/10.1007/s11920-015-0614-9.

2. Burger, J., et al. "A double-blinded, randomized, placebo-controlled sub-dissociative dose ketamine pilot study in the treatment of acute depression and suicidality in a military emergency department setting." *Military Medicine* 181, no. 10 (October 2016): 1195–99. https://doi.org/10.7205/MILMED-D-15-00431.

3. Fan, W., et al. "Ketamine rapidly relieves acute suicidal ideation in cancer patients: a randomized controlled clinical trial." *Oncotarget* 8, no. 2 (January 10, 2017): 2356–60. https://doi.org/10.18632/oncotarget.13743.

4. Price, R. B., et al. "Effects of ketamine on explicit and implicit suicidal cognition: a randomized controlled trial in treatment-resistant depression." *Depression and Anxiety* 31, no. 4 (April 2014): 335–43. https://doi.org/10.1002/da.22253.

5. Ballard, E. D., et al. "Anhedonia as a clinical correlate of suicidal thoughts in clinical ketamine trials." *Journal of Affective Disorders* 218 (August 15, 2017): 195–200. https://doi.org/10.1016/j.jad.2017.04.057.

6. Wilkowska, A., Szałach, Ł. P., and Cubała W. J. "Gut microbiota in depression: a focus on ketamine." *Frontiers in Behavioral Neuroscience* 15 (June 23, 2021): 693362. https://doi.org/10.3389/fnbeh.2021.693362.

7. Feder, A., et al. "A randomized controlled trial of repeated ketamine administration for chronic posttraumatic stress disorder." *American Journal of Psychiatry* 178, no. 2 (February 1, 2021): 193–202. https://doi.org/10.1176/appi.ajp.2020.20050596.

8. Dakwar, E., and Nunes, E. V. "New directions in medication-facilitated behavioral treatment for substance use disorders." *Current Psychiatry Reports* 18, no. 7 (July 2016): 64. https://doi.org/10.1007/s11920-016-0703-4.

9. Ezquerra-Romano, I., et al. "Ketamine for the treatment of addiction: Evidence and potential mechanisms." *Neuropharmacology* 142 (2018): 72–82. https://doi.org/10.1016/j.neuropharm.2018.01.017.

10. Dakwar, E., et al. "A single ketamine infusion combined with mindfulness-based behavioral modification to treat cocaine dependence: a randomized clinical trial." *American Journal of Psychiatry* 176, no. 11 (November 1, 2019): 923–30. https://doi.org/10.1176/appi.ajp.2019.18101123. Krupitsky, E., et al. "Ketamine psychotherapy for heroin addiction: immediate effects and two-year follow-up." *Journal of Substance Abuse Treatment* 23, no. 4 (December 2002): 273–83. https://doi.org/10.1016/s0740-5472(02)00275-1. Yoon, G., Petrakis, I. L., and Krystal, J. H. "Association of combined naltrexone and ketamine with depressive symptoms in a case series of patients with depression and alcohol use disorder." *JAMA Psychiatry* 76, no. 3 (2019): 337–38. https://doi.org/10.1001/jamapsychiatry.2018.3990.

11. Williams, N. R., et al. "Attenuation of antidepressant effects of ketamine by opioid receptor antagonism." *American Journal of Psychiatry* 175, no. 12 (August 2018): 1205–15. https://doi.org/10.1176/appi.ajp.2018.18020138.

12. Yoon, Petrakis, and Krystal. *JAMA Psychiatry* 76, 337–338.

13. Martinotti, G., et al. "Therapeutic potentials of ketamine and esketamine in obsessive-compulsive disorder (OCD), substance use disorders (SUD) and eating disorders (ED): A review of the current literature." *Brain Sciences* 11, no. 7 (June 27, 2021): 856. https://doi.org/10.3390/brainsci11070856. Matteo, M., et al. "The use of esketamine in comorbid treatment resistant depression and obsessive compulsive disorder following extensive pharmacogenomic testing: A case report." *Annals of General Psychiatry* 20, no. 1 (September 16, 2021): 43. https://doi.org/10.1186/s12991-021-00365-z. Thompson, S. L., et al. "Ketamine induces immediate and delayed alterations of OCD-like behavior." *Psychopharmacology* (Berlin) 237, no. 3 (March 2020): 627–38. https://doi.org/10.1007/s00213-019-05397-8.

14. Mills, I. H., et al. "Treatment of compulsive behaviour in eating disorders with intermittent ketamine infusions." *QJM: An International Journal of Medicine* 91, no. 7 (July 1998): 493–503. https://doi.org/10.1093/qjmed/91.7.493.

15. De Kock, M., Loix, S., and Lavand'homme, P. "Ketamine and peripheral inflammation." *CNS Neurosciences & Therapeutics* 19, no. 6 (June 2013): 403–10. https://doi.org/10.1111/cns.12104.

16. Lauritsen, C., et al. "Intravenous ketamine for subacute treatment of refractory chronic migraine: A case series." *Journal of Headache Pain* 17, no. 1 (December 2016): 106. https://doi.org/10.1186/s10194-016-0700-3.

17. Zitek, T., et al. "A comparison of headache treatment in the emergency department: prochlorperazine versus ketamine." *Annals of Emergency Medicine* 71, no. 3 (March 2018): 369–77. e1. https://doi.org/10.1016/j.annemergmed.2017.08.063.

18. Bell, J. D. "In vogue: Ketamine for neuroprotection in acute neurologic injury." *Anesthesia & Analgesia* 124, no. 4 (April 2017): 1237–43. https://doi.org/10.1213 /ANE.0000000000001856. Schiavone, S., et al. "Antidepressant drugs for beta amyloid-induced depression: A new standpoint?" *Progress in Neuro-Psychopharmacology and Biological Psychiatry* 78 (August 1, 2017): 114–122. https://doi.org/10.1016/j .pnpbp.2017.05.004.

19. Li, H., et al. "Ketamine suppresses proliferation and induces ferroptosis and apoptosis of breast cancer cells by targeting the KAT5/GPX4 axis." *Biochemical and Biophysical Research Communications* 585 (December 31, 2021): 111–16. https://doi.org/10.1016 /j.bbrc.2021.11.029.

CHAPTER 6

1. aan het Rot, M., et al. "Safety and efficacy of repeated-dose intravenous ketamine for treatment-resistant depression." *Biological Psychiatry* 67, no. 2 (2010): 139–45. https://doi.org/10.1016/j.biopsych.2009.08.038.

CHAPTER 11

1. Clements, J. A., Nimmo, W.S., and Grant, I.S. "Bioavailability, pharmacokinetics, and analgesic activity of ketamine in humans." *Journal of Pharmaceutical Sciences* 71, no. 5 (May 1982): 539–42. https://doi.org/10.1002/jps.2600710516.

2. Ibid. Rolan, P., et al. "The absolute bioavailability of racemic ketamine from a novel sublingual formulation." *British Journal of Clinical Pharmacology* 77, no. 6 (June 2014): 1011–16. https://doi.org/10.1111/bcp.12264.

3. World Health Organization. "Ataractic and hallucinogenic drugs in psychiatry; report of a study group." World Health Organization Technical Report Series 58, no. 152 (1958): 1–72.

4. Leary, T. *Flashbacks: An Autobiography* (Los Angeles: Tarcher, 1983).

5. Shemesh, A., et al. "Affective response to architecture—investigating human reaction to spaces with different geometry." *Architectural Science Review* 60, no. 2 (2017): 116–25. https://doi.org/10.1080/00038628.2016.1266597.

CHAPTER 14

1. Russ Harris, ACT with Love: Stop Struggling, Reconcile Differences, and Strengthen Your Relationship... with Acceptance and Commitment Therapy (Oakland, CA: New Harbinger Publications, 2009).

CHAPTER 15

1. Sessa, B. "From sacred plants to psychotherapy: The history and re-emergence of psychedelics in medicine." *European Neuropsychopharmacology* 17, supp. no 4 (2007): S215–S216. https://doi.org/10.1016/S0924-977X(07)70278-X.

2. Yalom, I. D., and Leszcz, M. *The Theory and Practice of Group Psychotherapy*. (New York: Basic Books, 2005).

3. Dames, S., Kryskow, P., and Watler, C. "A cohort-based case report: The impact of ketamine-assisted psychotherapy embedded in a community of practice framework for healthcare providers with PTSD and depression." *Frontiers in Psychiatry* (2022). https://doi.org/10.3389/fpsyt.2022.962882.

4. Yalom, I. D., and Leszcz, M. "The Therapeutic Factors." In *The Theory and Practice of Group Psychotherapy*, 6th ed. (New York: Basic Books, 2021), 15.

INDEX

ABOUT THE AUTHORS

Dr. Mike Dow is a *New York Times* best-selling author and has been dubbed America's go-to therapist. As a brain health, relationship, and addiction expert, Dr. Mike has hosted hit therapy-based shows on several networks including TLC, Disney+, E!, and VH1. He was part of Dr. Oz's core team of experts on *The Dr. Oz Show*, is a recurring guest co-host on *The Doctors*, and has made regular appearances on *Today, The Talk, Rachael Ray, Wendy Williams, Nancy Grace, Dr. Drew on Call*, and Canada's *The Marilyn Denis Show*. He has an M.S. in marriage and family therapy, a Psy.D. in psychology, and a Ph.D. in clinical sexology. Dr. Mike trained in Mindfulness-Based Cognitive Therapy (MBCT) at the University of California, Los Angeles, advanced clinical hypnosis with the American Society of Clinical Hypnosis (ASCH), and completed the Professionals in Residence program at the renowned Betty Ford Center. He is a graduate of the University of Southern California where he was a presidential scholar, and currently practices Ketamine-Assisted Psychotherapy at Field Trip. You can usually find Mike with his husband, Chris, and their dog, Emmett, in Los Angeles.

Connect with Dr. Mike at:

Website: drmikedow.com

Social: @drmikedow

Ronan Levy is an entrepreneur, author, and subject of *The Ordinary Trip* documentary, as well as a thought leader on the social and cultural impacts of the emerging psychedelic renaissance. Inspired by his own journey of personal growth, Ronan believes that you should never hesitate to trade your cow for a handful of magic beans. A lawyer by training, Ronan started his career as a securities lawyer at Blake, Cassels & Graydon LLP but left after realizing he was much too creative for the law profession. Since then, Ronan has helped launch businesses across a number of industries, from gold to cannabis, and most recently in psychedelics, where he co-founded Field Trip, a global leader in the development and delivery of psychedelic therapies. Ronan is also the host of the leading psychedelic podcast, *Field Tripping*, and co-author of *The Trip Journal*. When not being thoroughly incorrigible, Ronan lives in Toronto with his wife and two children.

Connect with Ronan at:

Website: fieldtriphealth.com

Social: @fieldtriphealth

Hay House Titles of Related Interest

YOU CAN HEAL YOUR LIFE, the movie,
starring Louise Hay & Friends
(available as an online streaming video)
www.hayhouse.com/louise-movie

THE SHIFT, the movie,
starring Dr. Wayne W. Dyer
(available as an online streaming video)
www.hayhouse.com/the-shift-movie

***

*CONNECTED FATES, SEPARATE DESTINIES: Using Family
Constellations Therapy to Recover from Inherited Stories and Trauma,*
by Marine Sélénée

TRAUMA: Healing Your Past to Find Freedom Now,
by Pedram Shojai, O.M.D. and Nick Polizzi

*SOUL JOURNEYING: Shamanic Tools for Finding Your Destiny
and Recovering Your Spirit,* by Alberto Villoldo

*BREAKING THE HABIT OF BEING YOURSELF: How to
Lose Your Mind and Create a New One,* by Dr. Joe Dispenza

All of the above are available at www.hayhouse.co.uk

***

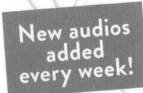

CONNECT WITH
HAY HOUSE
ONLINE

🌐 hayhouse.co.uk   **f** @hayhouse

📷 @hayhouseuk   🐦 @hayhouseuk

▶ @hayhouseuk   ♪ @hayhouseuk

Find out all about our latest books & card decks • Be the first to know about exclusive discounts • Interact with our authors in live broadcasts • Celebrate the cycle of the seasons with us • Watch free videos from your favourite authors • Connect with like-minded souls

'The gateways to wisdom and knowledge
are always open.'

Louise Hay